D0082635

Personality Disorder

Forensic Focus Series

This series, edited by Gwen Adshead, takes the field of Forensic Psychotherapy as its focal point, offering a forum for the presentation of theoretical and clinical issues. It embraces such influential neighbouring disciplines as language, law, literature, criminology, ethics and philosophy, as well as psychiatry and psychology, its established progenitors. Gwen Adshead is Consultant Forensic Psychotherapist and Lecturer in Forensic Psychotherapy at Broadmoor Hospital.

Forensic Focus 29

Personality Disorder
The Definitive Reader

Edited by Gwen Adshead and Caroline Jacob

Jessica Kingsley Publishers
London and Philadelphia

First published in 2009
by Jessica Kingsley Publishers
116 Pentonville Road
London N1 9JB, UK
and
400 Market Street, Suite 400
Philadelphia, PA 19106, USA

www.jkp.com

Library of Congress Cataloging in Publication Data
Personality disorder : the definitive reader / edited by Gwen Adshead and Caroline Jacob.
    p. ; cm.
Includes bibliographical references.
ISBN 978-1-84310-640-1 (pb : alk. paper)
1. Personality disorders. I. Adshead, Gwen. II. Jacob, Caroline.
[DNLM: 1. Personality Disorders--Collected Works. WM 190 P4666 2009]
RC554.P465 2009
616.85'81--dc22

                                                    2008022590

British Library Cataloguing in Publication Data
A CIP catalogue record for this book is available from the British Library

ISBN 978 1 84310 640 1

Printed and bound in Great Britain by
Athenaeum Press, Gateshead, Tyne and Wear

Dedicated to the memory of Murray Cox,
Consultant Psychotherapist in Broadmoor Hospital
between 1975 and 1997.
We miss him still.

I'm blind because I see too much, so I study by a dark lamp

(Cox 1995)

Acknowledgements

This book would not have been possible without the encouragement and support of Nick Benefield, practical and editorial advice from Jessica Kingsley Publishers and the patience and creativity of Pauline Watson, PA to the London Psychotherapy Service. Our grateful thanks to all of them, and to all colleagues who have supported us in our work with patients with personality disorders.

Contents

Part III Treatment and Management

Introduction

The Personality Disorder Reader is intended to act as a resource for all staff working with personality disorder. There has been a huge increase in services for people with personality disorder, and there has been a commensurate increase in the need for education and training in this area for all staff disciplines. We ourselves have benefited from reading papers about personality disorder during our training, so we took the view that it would be helpful for colleagues to have a collection of papers that focused on the complexities of working with patients with personality disorder.

In putting together this collection, we sought recommendations from a wide range of colleagues: senior teachers, diploma students in forensic psychiatry and psychotherapy, service users, and colleagues in practice. There are a mixture of classic and more recent papers; also a mixture of theoretical orientations. We think this is appropriate because personality disorder is such a complicated condition that it requires a multidisciplinary approach. We also think that this mixture of papers reflects the fact that our knowledge of the field of personality disorder continues to increase and we cannot afford to ignore any possible contribution.

The papers are roughly divided into sections that deal with aetiology, clinical presentation and professional responses. The papers may be used as a resource for training, a supervision aid and an easily accessible 'reminder' to us about the complexities of the work we do. Between sections we have set out some questions that could form the basis of journal clubs or reflective practice sessions. We hope very much that the Reader will be practically useful for all colleagues working in the field.

REFERENCES

Cox, M. (1995) Special hospitals as agents of change: psychotherapy at Broadmoor. *Criminal Justice Matters*, *21*: 10–11.

Part I

Theory: Aetiology and Psychopathology

1

The Relationship Between Severity of Personality Disorder and Certain Adverse Childhood Influences[*]

Michael Craft, Geoffrey Stephenson
and Clive Granger
1964

· ·

Editors' reflections

It remains puzzling why some individuals who experience significant childhood trauma appear to emerge with minimal personality disturbance whilst others present with severe personality disorder. In acknowledging that childhood experiences may predispose individuals to developing personality disorder, the following paper aims to extend the link further. It considers the hypothesis that the degree of personality disturbance may be correlated to particular adverse childhood events, both in type and frequency of exposure.

· ·

[*] Originally published in *British Journal of Psychiatry*, *110*, 392–396. Reprinted here by permission of The Royal College of Psychiatrists.

INTRODUCTION

This paper reports the result of an investigation into the hypothesis that severity of personality disturbance is positively related to the frequency of certain early adverse childhood influences.

The relationship between early adverse childhood influences, particularly maternal separation, and later delinquency or personality disturbance has been the subject of increasing numbers of studies in this century, but the above hypothesis does not appear to have been tested. Barbara Wootton (1959), in her critical survey of studies on maternal separation, claims that results show only that 'as things are at present, children have a better chance of finding dependable love in families than in institutions'. It remains to be proved, she states, that maternal separation per se is a 'pathogenic factor' as Ainsworth and Bowlby (1954) would claim. Her conclusion explicitly rejects Ainsworth and Bowlby's fundamental postulates: 'That damage (caused by maternal separation) is lifelong or irreversible, that maternal deprivation is a major factor in criminal behaviour, or that the younger the child the greater the risk, all these must be regarded as quite unproven hypotheses' (p.156). Wootton (1959) finds the evidence for a link between maternal separation and actual delinquency particularly weak. No study, she claims, has shown unequivocally that delinquents receive more than their due of maternal separation, or that separated children are disproportionately delinquent, whilst some studies suggest that the maternal separation hypothesis should be rejected (Andry 1959; Lewis 1954). Certain work however (Brandon 1960; Holman 1953; Lewis 1954), does suggest that paternal separation is perhaps equally important, but no convincing relationship between paternal absence and later development of delinquency or psychopathy has yet been demonstrated.

Recently Naess (1962) has noted that the incidence of mother-separation during childhood varied markedly in the different groups of delinquents investigated by him, and has suggested that this was related to the unequal severity of delinquency in the groups studied, but no detailed comparisons are given. Illegitimacy, usually denoting absence of a father, and often associated with other adverse factors such as maternal hostility, has been repeatedly shown to be correlated with maladjustment (Lewis 1954; Pringle 1961) and psychopathy (Rowe 1931). Pringle (1961) found 14 per cent of boys and 17 per cent of girls in 2,593 maladjusted children in residential schools to be illegitimate compared with a 4–7 per cent national average. In Lewis' (1954) study of 500 Kentish children removed from home, of whom 76 per cent were maladjusted, 23 per cent were illegitimate. Illegitimacy was also noted to correlate with reconvictions in a recent series of 100 admissions to a psychopathic unit, a high proportion of the illegitimate belonging to the more severe approved school transfers in the series (Craft et al. 1964).

The incidence of patients giving a positive history of previous brain damage has repeatedly been shown to be high in groups of delinquents and psychopaths (Rogers et al. 1956; Rowe 1931; Naess 1962; Stafford-Clark and Taylor 1949). Although some of these early papers are very vague in their definitions, specific examples of temporal and frontal lobe damage make it clear that damage to particular areas of the brain can be responsible for certain personality disorders (Erikson 1945; Pygott and Street 1960; Terzian et al. 1955).

Many other early adverse childhood experiences have been noted by recent investigators, notably the Gluecks, but maternal and paternal separation, illegitimacy and brain damage have been used in this study, which follows from one published earlier (Craft 1959), partly because with these factors patients' accounts can be readily checked from their documents, and partly because this was intended as a pilot study.

METHOD USED TO TEST INITIAL HYPOTHESIS

As a result of the activities of the Balderton Psychopathic Unit (Craft 1959; Craft 1960; Craft 1961; Craft et al. 1962) the authors were brought into contact with six groups of males, all of whom were over I.Q. 60 on testing. Firstly, there were 76 Special Hospital patients in Rampton, Moss Side or Broadmoor Hospitals. These contained 21 patients described previously (Craft 1959) who had been transferred to these hospitals on the grounds of extreme behaviour disorder, 12 youths with psychopathic disorder aged 17–25 within Rampton in 1961, and 43 male admissions from 1960–61 to Moss Side. As each series was made up of consecutive casenotes and was unselected except for I.Q. there is not felt to be any bias in adding them together.

The second and third groups consisted of 100 consecutive admissions for delinquency with mental disorder to the Balderton Unit (Craft et al. 1962) together with one extra patient included in a further series (Craft et al. 1964). These were divided into two groups, Balderton 'A' comprising 21 approved school transfers and Balderton 'B', 80 further patients mainly on probation.

The fourth group studied consisted of all 28 boys resident at a Junior Approved School during the winter 1960–61, whilst the fifth group comprised the 68 boys resident at an Intermediate Approved School in May, 1962. One of us was consultant psychiatrist to both these schools, which contained predominantly Northern English children. Group six consisted of 24 boys aged 15–23 connected with a Nottingham youth club in an area from which many of the Balderton psychopaths came and to which many were discharged. These youths were selected as being those prepared to be subjects for a research project.

Eighty-eight per cent, of patients were studied by one of us (M.C.), 12 per cent by the other (G.S.) using the same defined criteria. An additional group of 50 Grammar and 50 Secondary Modern schoolboys aged 15 was studied by one of us (G.S.); in this group only part of the above data were obtained, and are therefore appended at the end of the results.

To investigate the hypothesis, the groups were placed in order of severity of behaviour disturbance. There was little doubt that the Special Hospital patients contained the most severe psychopaths, for a substantial proportion were in this category under the Mental Health Act, or that those who had had to be transferred to Balderton from Approved Schools on the grounds of behaviour disturbance should come second. It was decided to place the probationers in Balderton third, for these youths had been sent by courts to Balderton rather than to Approved Schools on the ground of psychopathic traits, and the observed level of behaviour disturbance came above the observed level of the Approved schoolboys. It was more difficult to place the youngsters in the Junior Approved School, for although the disturbances shown by these boys were extreme they were also most changeable at this age. The Intermediate Approved schoolboys were found to contain many 'simple' situational delinquents from big cities; and so these and the Nottingham youth club boys came fifth and sixth. The Secondary Modern and Grammar schoolboy group is seventh, but probably contains bias for social class and intelligence.

Having placed the groups in order, the initial hypothesis was checked by using adverse childhood influences chosen to be as objective as possible. These consisted of periods of a year or more of absence of mother or father during childhood up to 10 years old; illegitimacy; and brain damage defined as previous encephalitis or meningitis, properly documented birth injury, or road or civil accident causing hospital admission and unconsciousness for longer than an hour. These factors were analysed from the casenotes and checked from other documents, and direct from the patients, most of whom were under the senior author's care.

RESULTS

In this section the groups are ranked according to the frequency of the adverse factors found from casenotes and personal examination. The rankings found are compared with the rankings predicted on the ground of severity of personality disorder. The seven groups, ranked in expected order of least severity of personality disturbance, are shown in Table I.

Table I			
	Average Age	*No. in Sample*	*Predicted Rank*
Secondary Modern and Grammar schoolboys	15.5	100	1
Youth Club	18.7	24	2
Intermediate Approved School	15.2	68	3
Junior Approved School	11.3	28	4
Balderton B	23.0	80	5
Balderton A	19.6	21	6
Special Hospitals	26.0	76	7

Table II shows the results of ranking the groups according to the proportions having no parental deprivation (col. A), no illegitimacy (col. B), no brain damage (col. C), and none of these (col. D). There is strong evidence of a connection between severity of delinquency and some combination of parental deprivation, illegitimacy; and brain damaged. The predicted rank and that in column D are identical, and the ranking of column A agrees significantly with the predicted ranking (at 99 per cent, confidence level using Spearman's rank correlation test).

In Table III the average number of years of absence of each boy's mother and father during 0–10 years of age is listed, together with rankings alongside. The table suggests that the duration of absence might also contribute to a significant ranking, but in fact ranking only becomes significant when the average duration of absence of both mother and father is summed. Such a sum is of doubtful validity, since where both parents are absent the absence of one is probably related to the absence of the other. Dividing the duration of absence into that occurring from 0–5 and 5–10 years of age, the average absence was equally distributed between the two periods. Neither appears to be the more important in relation to results.

Table II

	A No Parental Deprivation			B No Illegitimacy			C No Brain Damage			D No Parental Deprivation, Illegitimacy or Brain Damage		
	No.	Proportion	Rank	No.	Proportion	Rank	No.	Proportion	Rank	No.	Proportion	Rank
Schoolboys	91	0.91	1	*		*	93	0.93	1	85*	0.85	1
Youth Club	18	0.75	2	23	0.96	1	20	0.83	4	15	0.63	2
Intermediate Approved School	42	0.62	3	55	0.81	4	55	0.81	5	35	0.52	3
Junior Approved School	12	0.43	5	22	0.79	5	24	0.86	5	9	0.32	4
Balderton B	37	0.46	4	69	0.86	2	64	0.90	6	24	0.30	5
Balderton A	6	0.28	7	14	0.67	6	18	0.86	2	5	0.23	6
Special Hospitals	29	0.35	6	63	0.83	3	51	0.69	7	16	0.19	7

* Illegitimacy was not ascertained for the schoolboy group, so that column D does not contain this information. However when the original data sheets were used to combine information for parental deprivation and brain damage alone for the seven groups, the schoolboy group remained first in rank order.

Table III

	Predicted Rank	I Average Years Father Absent	Rank	II Average Years Mother Absent	Rank
Youth Club	1	0.67	1	0.54	1
Intermediate Approved School	2	1.95	2	0.75	2
Junior Approved School	3	3.25	4	2.22	5
Balderton B	4	2.70	3	1.14	3
Balderton A	5	4.24	6	1.95	4
Special Hospitals	6	3.52	5	3.08	6

The illegitimacy rate amongst the delinquents seems high, so the proportion of illegitimacy in all groups excluding the youth club was compared with the appropriate population illegitimacy rate. Forty-five (16 per cent) of the 275 boys in the five delinquent groups are illegitimate. Taking the proportion legitimate in the total (relevant) population as 9 per cent (i.e. high upper bound), a large sample proportions test still rejects the hypothesis that the proportion of delinquents who are illegitimate is the same as for the whole population, at a very high significance level (p.<003).

Verification of the youth club rankings is found in the data obtained from the 100 schoolboys who were a cross-section of all fourth-year boys in two State schools. Full data were obtained with respect to brain damage and parental deprivation from the boys themselves and their school records and showed that 91 per cent (0.93) had no history of brain damage. These proportions are less than shown by any of the other groups, including the youth club, but because data were not obtained for illegitimacy and because many of the Grammar schoolboys were of higher social class than those in other groups, the results must be considered with caution. They are in keeping with the stated hypothesis.

COMMENTS AND CONCLUSIONS

The hypothesis that among groups of delinquents and psychopaths severity of personality disorder is positively related to the frequency of certain adverse environmental influence is supported.

It might be objected that as the groups are of different ages, particular social class, economic affluence or separation due to the war might be relevant to the ranking, particularly of parental absence and illegitimacy. However, these influences would tend to place the youth club group lower in the list of predicted rank order, whilst increased war illegitimacy would tend to place the two Approved Schools groups higher, for, being born post-war they should have least parental separation and illegitimacy.

Social class has obvious associations with illegitimacy and parental desertion, and possible bias due to this must be assessed. Additional data for social class were available for the Special Hospital group, none of whom had parents in the Registrar-General classes 1 and 2; the Balderton groups with 10 parents in classes 1 and 2 (10 per cent) and the youth club, 15 (63 per cent) of whom had parents in class 3, and 9 (37 per cent) in class 4. In the youth club group there were no parents in classes 1, 2 and 5. As Gittins (1952), Stott (1950) and others have shown, Approved schoolboys very rarely have parents in social classes 1 and 2. Only the schoolboy group would appear to show a bias by way of social class.

Liability to brain damage presumably rises as age advances and is certainly highest among the oldest Special Hospital group. It is however, second highest in the youngest group, and there is no good reason for supposing there is differential admission here, except on the grounds of resultant disturbed behaviour.

It is important to note that, although this study suggests a relationship between severity of disorder and frequency and degree of certain early adverse factors, in particular of parental separation, it does not mean that such influences are aetiological factors in the development of psychopathic personality. It is quite possible that actual maternal and paternal absences are minor factors in aetiology, it being the adverse parental attitudes and material circumstances contingent upon prolonged absences that exert the important effect on the developing child.

Our study used a very simple ranking of different groups, determined by fairly clear clinical considerations that few would dispute. The procedure is only justifiable as a pilot study, and further research is in progress in Wales to check the hypothesis in a different cultural area and to assess the importance of other early adverse childhood influences, such as parental attitudes and under-privilege, in their contribution to clinically defined degrees of personality disturbance.

ACKNOWLEDGEMENTS

We are grateful to the Medical Superintendents of Rampton, Moss Side and Broadmoor for ready help and permission to visit their hospitals and see patients and case histories, and to the headmasters of the Approved, Grammar and Secondary Modern schools.

REFERENCES

Ainsworth, M.D. and Bowlby, J. (1954) Research strategy in the study of mother-child separation. *Courier*, 3.

Andry, R.G. (1959) *Delinquency and Parental Pathology*. London: Methuen and Co.

Brandon, S. (1960) Epidemiological study of maladjustment in childhood. M.D. Thesis, Durham.

Craft, M. (1959) Personality disorder and dullness. *Lancet*, 1, 856.

Craft, M. (1960) A psychopathic unit and its community setting. *Journal of the Mentally Subnormal*, 6, 23.

Craft, M. (1961) A psychopathic unit at Balderton. *Bethlem Royal and Maudsley Gazette*, 4, 214.

Craft, M., Fabisch, W., Stephenson, G., Burnand, G. and Kerridge, D. (1962) 100 admissions to a psychopathic unit. *Journal of Mental Sciences*, 108, 504.

Craft, M., Stephenson, G. and Granger, C. (1964) A controlled trial of authoritarian and self-governing regimes with adolescent psychopaths. *American Journal of Orthopsychiatry*, 34, 543–554.

Erikson, T.C. (1945) Erotomania as an expression of cortinal discharge. *Archives of Neurology and Psychiatry*, 53, 226.

Gittins, J. (1952) *Approved Schoolboys*. H.M.S.O.

Holman, P. (1953) Some factors in the aetiology of maladjusted children. *Journal of Mental Science*, 99, 657.

Lewis, H. (1954) *Deprived Children*. London: O.U.P. for the Nuffield Foundation.

Naess, S. (1962) Mother separation and delinquency. *British Journal of Criminology*, 2, 361.

Pringle, K. (1961) *The incidence of some supposedly adverse family conditions. British Journal of Educational Psychiatry*, 31, 183.

Pygott, F. and Street, D.F. (1960) Unsuspected treatable organic dementia. *Lancet*, 1, 1371.

Rogers, M.E., Lilenfeld, A.H. and Pasamanick, B. (1956) *Prenatal and Paranatal Factors in the Development of Childhood Behaviour Disorders*. Washington, DC: Johns Hopkins University.

Rowe, A.W. (1931) A possible endocrine factor in the behaviour problems of the young. *American Journal of Orthopsychiatry*, 1, 451.

Stafford-Clark, D. and Taylor, F.H. (1949) Clinical and EEG studies on prisoners charged with murder. *Journal of Neurology, Neurosurgery and Psychiatry*, 12, 325.

Stott, D.H. (1950) *Delinquency and Human Nature*. Fife: Carnegie Trust.

Terzian, H. and Dalle Ore, G. (1955) Syndrome of Klüver and Bucy: Reproduced in man by bilateral removal of temporal lobes. *Neurology*, 5, 373–380.

Thompson, G.M. (1945) Psychiatric factors influencing learning. *Journal of Nervous and Mental Diseases*, 101, 347.

Wootton, B. (1959) *Social Science and Social Pathology*. London: Allen and Unwin.

2

Care-Eliciting Behaviour in Man[*]

Scott Henderson, M.D.[1]
1974

. . . .

Editors' reflections

The following paper was published thirty years ago, and is one of the first papers to make an explicit link between attachment theory and general psychiatry. It is also exceptionally helpful because it reframes troubling behaviours that upset health care professionals as having meaning for service users, in terms of early experiences with their carers. This means that we can understand people with personality disorders as people who do not know how to elicit care effectively from others; and indeed, tend to elicit care in coercive or threatening ways. Such an understanding allows us to make links between this paper and more recent research on attachment as involving both care-giving and care-eliciting. Thanks to Dr Christopher Bass for drawing our attention to this paper.

. . . .

Abstract

The concept of care-eliciting behaviour is proposed as an essential part of the phenomenon of attachment. The origins of this behaviour in man are examined in terms of both ontogenesis and phylogenesis. The relevance of the behaviour for species advantage is considered. Finally, it is suggested that morbid manifestations of care-eliciting constitute a number of psychiatric disorders previously considered to be unrelated.

[*]   Originally published in *Journal of Nervous and Mental Disorder*, 15, 3, 172–181. Reprinted here by permission of Lippincott Williams & Wilkins.

INTRODUCTION

> It will be necessary to search for the roots and the manifestations of our inner lives everywhere: In the souls of children, of primitive men, of animals. Furthermore, it will be necessary to establish to what degree lost emotions of the individual and of the phylogenetic past are reborn in illness (Kraepelin 1971, p.7).

The determinants of social behaviour are of central importance to clinical psychiatry. The most fundamental of these is dependence, yet as Parens and Saul (1971) have recently emphasized, the subject has not yet occupied a place in the literature commensurate with its importance. For a concept so widely used in everyday clinical work, it is surprising that the word dependence does not appear in the index of the collected works of Freud (1946). A detailed examination of dependence, as expressed in primary affectional bonding, came with the work of Bowlby (1969, 1973). The present paper is an attempt to develop two particular aspects of the subject: firstly, the phylogenetic basis of dependence in adulthood; and secondly, its pathology, where it is either present in excess or is manifest in deviant ways by adults. These two aspects are interrelated, since pathological manifestations of dependence reflect only the deviant expression of a phylogenetically important behaviour.

Bowlby, in the second volume of his work on attachment and loss, says:

> Perhaps no terms are used more frequently in the clinical literature than 'dependent' and 'overdependent'. A child who tends to be clinging, an adolescent reluctant to leave home, a wife or husband who maintains close contact with mother, an invalid who demands company, all these and others are likely sooner or later to be described with one of these words. Always in their use there is an aura of disapproval, of disparagement (1973, p.212).

In his previous volume, Bowlby (1969) had recommended that the word 'dependency' be replaced by the term 'attachment', mainly because of its failure to reflect the true bi-directional nature of the relationship and its pejorative connotations. For the purpose of describing that part of dependency or attachment behaviour that elicits care from another, the present author proposes the term 'care-eliciting'. This may be defined as a pattern of activity on the part of one individual, which evokes from another responses that give comfort. The latter may take many forms such as providing close body contact or, at a more complex level, the expression of concern, esteem, or affection through language. The concept of care-eliciting behaviour may prove of considerable theoretical and clinical usefulness if, on the basis of ethological principles, it assists in the recognition of aetiology in the neuroses and behaviour disorders, if it provides hypotheses about populations at risk and if it points the way to effective treatment.

PHYLOGENETIC ORIGINS

The emergence of ethology as a science which observes rigorous standards has encouraged a few workers to look to it for help in understanding human behaviour (Bowlby 1969, 1973, Hamburg 1971). Tiger (1969) describes this attractively as an attempt to link 'the microhistory of social sciences to the macrohistory of species biology'. So far, most attention has been paid to aggression, particularly in infrahuman primates (De Vore 1963, Hamburg 1971, Lorenz 1966) and to the phenomena associated with primary affectional bonding (Harlow 1960, Harlow and Harlow 1966, Hinde and Spencer-Booth 1971). Less prominently, Scott (1969, p.777–790), a distinguished behavioural scientist, has given an account of what he calls 'et-epimeletic behaviour' in birds and mammals. He describes this category of behaviour as 'having the function of calling or signalling for help and attention' (p.778). The possibility that this ethological formulation may have relevance for clinical psychiatry holds considerable appeal and was the original stimulus for the arguments developed in this paper.

Hamburg (1968, p.42) has argued that certain primate species 'are more likely than others to provide interesting leads that stimulate research in the contemporary human species from an evolutionary perspective'. In rhesus monkeys under laboratory conditions, Harlow and his group (Harlow 1960, Harlow and Harlow 1966) described the infant monkey's preference for 'contact comfort' obtained from terry-towelling mother surrogates and how this comfort was particularly sought when the infant was presented with frightening stimuli. Such observations are of the greatest importance, but their limitation is that they refer only to the primary bonding process in the young and to attachment behaviour in the laboratory setting. For observing primate social behaviours such as care-eliciting and care-giving, the most suitable species is the chimpanzee, on which a body of ethological data has been collected by van Lawick-Goodall and her group in Tanzania (1968). It is here that one may begin to look for information on care-eliciting behaviour in infrahuman primates observed in the free-ranging state. In the chimpanzee infant, care-eliciting behaviour is directed principally at the mother and includes contact clinging, the 'hoo' whimper, screaming, and the pout face. Screaming is a powerful stimulus for the mother to return to the chimpanzee infant or to undertake cradling behaviour. In adult chimpanzees, grooming appears to be a prominent social activity by means of which anxiety and aggression are reduced. Two of van Lawick-Goodall's observations are of particular relevance to human interaction: She describes an adult female, Melissa, who 'rocked and whimpered if she was ignored and sometimes reached out to poke the male concerned, after this he often groomed her' (1968, p.263), and a male, Hugo, who would sometimes threaten his partner if the latter stopped grooming, shaking branches at him, staring and showing hair erection. These are essentially operant attachment behaviours, which bear a close resemblance to those shown by humans when dissatisfied with the attention being shown them.

Grooming in free-ranging chimpanzees usually takes place between pairs of individuals. In the mother–infant relationship, it plays little part at first but increases in frequency as the infant grows older. During the chimpanzee's childhood and adolescence, grooming progressively extends from the mother to a wider social group. It seems reasonable to conclude from this that grooming in chimpanzees is a social behaviour, which is developmentally related to the attachment behaviour of chimpanzee infants. It is also the best-described example of care-eliciting and care-taking behaviour in nonhuman primates. Since it is important to have as good an understanding of this behaviour as of aggression because of its relevance to an understanding of human relationships, much attention should now be accorded to care-eliciting patterns in infrahuman species.

NORMAL CARE-ELICITING BEHAVIOUR IN MAN

In studying the ontogeny of care-eliciting in man, one is faced with the question: Is care-eliciting in the adult derived from the attachment behaviour of infancy? At present, one can offer only indirect evidence for the ontogency of dependence by trying to relate adult care-eliciting behaviour to the attachment behaviour of infants. The attachment behaviours, which are most common in infants and children, are crying, arm raising, clinging, and returning to mother (Bowlby 1969, 1973). Crying and arm raising are both powerful stimuli for adults to initiate comforting activities. These behaviours in infants are ubiquitous and appear to be largely independent of culture. As Konner (1972, p.293) says in his description of infant crying amongst the Zhun-Twasi in Africa, 'it is the same intensely unpleasant sound, the one which one wants to hear stopped immediately'. These are therefore likely to be phylogenetically given behaviours shown by all children when exposed to the appropriate stimuli, with no learning component being present initially, although clearly the response by family and culture is likely to influence their subsequent pattern.

One might expect the attachment behaviour of infants to disappear with maturation since it is no longer biologically necessary for food and warmth. This does not appear to happen. The answer is that in earlier man and in infrahuman species, attachment behaviour in adults is likely to have carried considerable advantage for survival. The implications of the behaviour for modern man, in health and in illness still have to be explored. One would agree with Bowlby and Ainsworth (Bowlby 1973, Personal communication) that 'all the forms of attachment behaviour, including of course the care-eliciting behaviours, remain a normal part of the behavioural repertoire of humans throughout life'. During childhood and adolescence, the repertoire enlarges and relationships develop with others, strongly with one or two and less intensely with a larger number. Adults still cry when separated from loved ones, they cling when distressed and they sometimes find the close proximity of chosen others to be comforting. The importance of contact comfort in humans is illustrated by the observations of Hollender et al. (1970, p.387–390) on 'Correlates of the desire to be held in women'. These authors noted that many women, including well adjusted ones, use sexual intercourse as a means of having their partners hold them. It is the holding, itself developmentally primitive, from which these women derive pleasure, irrespective of their enjoyment of the sexual component of the encounter. In adults, many other behaviours are developed which elicit care: facial expressions or postures bespeaking sadness, minor somatic complaints and verbal requests for expressions of approbation, esteem, or love. Cultural factors seem to have a surprisingly limited influence on care-eliciting, being more likely to determine the degree to which it can be sanctioned than the form in which the behaviour is exhibited. This issue has been well illustrated by Doi (1969), who emphasizes that western psychiatrists tend to look upon dependency as an undesirable, infantile trait, whereas Indian writers such as Surya (1969, p.381) and others in Asia view it as behaviour which is wholly consonant with their culture and one which professionals would not seek to discourage. This is exemplified by the Japanese concept of 'amaeru', which Doi (1969) describes as an intransitive verb meaning 'to depend or presume upon another's love'. The word describes the relationship existing both between a mother and her infant and that, which, in Japan, may be socially sanctioned between two adults.

The following vignettes illustrate normal care-eliciting behaviour in western adults:

1. A young woman, recently married, finds that her husband is no longer according her the attention she requires. As initial acts of care-eliciting, she makes verbal requests for him to spend more time at home, to say frequently that he loves her, and to take her out occasionally. If such requests are ineffective, she goes on to use stronger signals, such as periods of sulking or weeping. This causes her husband some distress and he becomes much more solicitous toward her.

2. A husband finds that he has become of secondary importance in the household: his wife devotes most of her attention to the children, giving preference to *their* demands for her affection. In matters such as laundry, choice of food, and leisure activities, his preferences are overruled by the children's. He finally expresses his displeasure and pleads for his wife to return to her former affectionate self. Alternatively, he may become withdrawn and sullen at times. His wife then becomes concerned about him, briefly increasing her care-giving toward him. Occasionally, greatly to his wife's annoyance, he redirects his care-eliciting to other women. This pattern persists until the family cycle advances to allow him greater possession of his wife.

3. An elderly woman, accustomed to a satisfying role as a mother and wife, is bereaved of her husband. From a full life with many emotional rewards from her family and social contacts, she finds herself isolated and deprived of many previously satisfying sources, particularly her friends, her children, and her social status. In her grief, she initially sees life as being empty. She starts worrying unrealistically about money. By virtue of her own coping resources, she gradually re-establishes a circle of friends. Her attendance at church and at her general practitioner's both increases in frequency, and she regularly visits and telephones her offspring, perhaps more frequently than they would wish. At times she complains to her family of loneliness, when her facial expression and posture bespeak dejection and yearning.

For the young, the function of care-eliciting behaviour for species survival is self-evident: Only infants who successfully elicit care from their mothers will survive. As Bowlby (1969) has described in detail, the anaclitic situation in the infant not only ensures adequate nutrition and protection, but also establishes the capacity for pair-bonding in later life. In man, with the absence of oestrus as the specific period of female receptivity, a mechanism for the formation of strong and enduring heterosexual pair-bonds is likely to have conferred considerable reproductive advantage. Indeed, the continuation of the species itself may have been dependent on such a mechanism for males and females to come together and stay bonded for long periods. It is care-eliciting behaviour that is intimately concerned with this capacity to establish and maintain such affectional bonds and it is seen in its most developed state in our own species. Secondly, in addition to reproduction, care-eliciting has a function which is complementary to intraspecies aggression: it provides for the group a means of maintaining strong social bonds between all its members (Eibl-Eibesfeldt 1971). Van Lawick-Goodall (1968) comments that in infrahuman species, grooming is coming to be recognized as having a role in maintaining social relationships, while Sparks (1967) has suggested that social grooming is of greater importance the greater the rigidity of the social structure of a species. Care-eliciting behaviour has some claim to be regarded as having major biological importance.

PATHOLOGICAL CARE-ELICITING

The use of illness, both physical and psychiatric, for secondary gain or 'manipulation' of others is well recognized. Liberman and Raskin (1971) examined this closely in their behavioural formulation of depression. Freud in the 'Fragment of an Analysis of a Case of Hysteria' speaks of a woman for whom 'ill health will be her one weapon for maintaining her position. It will procure for her the care she longs for...it will compel him [her husband] to treat her with solicitude if she recovers, for otherwise a relapse will threaten' (1946, vol.3, p.55–56). By means of a theoretical model derived from ethology, it may now be possible to place under a single rubric a seemingly disparate group of disorders which have one common property: *They tend to occur when an individual perceives himself to be receiving insufficient caring behaviour from others.* These disorders may appropriately be called the 'care-eliciting syndromes'. A provisional list is shown in Table 1. This proposal earned the implication that these syndromes *are of the same order as or belong to the same behavioural system as the care-eliciting behaviour described above* and may have common origins in both ontogeny and phylogeny. The syndromes stand separately from normal care-eliciting behaviour only insofar as they are disruptive for the individual, or for others, or for both. It is well recognized in ethology that appetitive behaviours (such as care-eliciting) may have diverse motor patterns (Hinde 1970). In abnormal care-eliciting, instead of crying, clinging, or using verbal appeals, the individual uses other signals. These signals cause distress to himself and often to others, but their consequence is developmentally ancient; they bring important others closer.

TABLE 1 - Abnormal care-eliciting behaviour

A prominent component in:

Parasuicide

Neurotic depression

Conversion hysteria

Abnormal illness behaviour*

Anorexia nervosa

Shoplifting

Multiple illegitimate pregnancies

* Hypochondriasis, hysterical overlay, psychogenic pain, accident neurosis, dermatitis arte-facta, Munchausen syndrome, 'malingering'.

Parasuicide

The abnormal behaviour, which most closely lends itself to the care-eliciting paradigm is parasuicide (attempted suicide or acts of self-poisoning or self-injury). Stengel (1964) justifiably described this act as 'a cry for help', perhaps unwittingly referring to this developmentally primitive signal for care. The act of parasuicide rarely occurs in the absence of a recent dislocation in the individual's relationship with a significant other. Admittedly, the psychopathology is exceedingly complex in that the individual displays in one act a mixture of depression, despair, hostility, and a desire to be heeded (Kreitman *et al.* 1969, 1970). The motor act of parasuicide is only one component of a sequence of behaviours, each care-eliciting in character, but frequently not recognized as such by relatives or professionals alike. Following the act, one frequently cannot fail to be impressed at its effectiveness in modifying the behaviour and attitudes of those around the patient, including professionals. Within his own circle these modifications may be only temporary, but there is often the possibility in the minds of relatives that the act may be repeated (Rubinstein *et al.* 1958). One suspects that in some situations the act of parasuicide is at least equal to professional intervention in successfully altering the behaviour of others.

Neurotic depression

There is unlikely to be a rapid resolution of the unitary *vs.* binary views on depressive illness (Kendell 1969, Kiloh and Garside 1963, Paykel 1971). It is proposed here that some depressive behaviour is essentially care-eliciting. Children use crying to evoke the responses they wish. With maturity, other behaviours replace crying for the most part. A weeping adult represents a very powerful stimulus for others to approach and to offer comfort. The posture of a depressed person, with head bowed, a downward gaze, little eye contact, and the faces portraying sadness, comprises a strong stimulus for others to intervene. Neurotic depression falls into the care-eliciting group because it is a behavioural response to the withdrawal of sources of caring, the behaviour itself being an operant for caretaking to be reinstituted. Unless replaced by more adaptive behaviours, it may be maintained by the reinforcement provided by family and professionals. This formulation is wholly in accord with that of Liberman and Raskin (1971, p.519) who emphasized the operant function of depressive symptoms. They described how the depressed person 'generates very definite reactions from his interpersonal environment. These reactions are various forms of attention and may include sympathy, concern, interest, help-fulness, suggestions, and annoyance'. The implications of this formulation for treatment are considerable.

Conversion hysteria

It is becoming apparent to many writers, such as Slater (1965) and Guze (1907, p.491–498), that hysteria is not one disease but several. In addition, there are many models available to explain hysterical symptoms. As a minimum, there is the psychodynamic model, postulating the physical expression of unconscious conflict over a repressed wish. A second view is neurophysiologically based, and follows the finding of Lader and Sartorius (1968, p.490–495) that persons with conversion hysteria are very highly aroused. A third view is that taken by Szasz (1961) in which hysteria is seen as a form of primitive communication or protolanguage. This view is compatible with the present proposal to include many cases of conversion hysteria among the care-eliciting syndromes. Such cases are to be recognized by the presence of some serious interpersonal conflict, often involving a threat to the integrity of the pair-bond, affecting an individual who by reason of personality, intelligence or neurological disease is limited in his repertoire of alternative coping behaviours. Through the mechanism of dissociation, whether this is interpreted in psychological or neurophysiological terms, the individual develops a symptom, which has a profound effect on others and is commonly associated with a substantial increase in the amount of caring behaviour shown toward him.

Abnormal illness behaviour

This term was introduced by Pilowsky (1969, p.347–351) to denote an apparently heterogeneous group of clinical disorders, the main ones being hypochondriasis, psychogenic pain, hysterical overlay, compensation neurosis, 'malingering' and the Munchausen syndrome. Abnormal illness behaviour is defined as the persistence of an inappropriate mode of perceiving, evaluating, and acting in relation to one's health. Special attention will be focused here on hypochondriasis. Kreitman *et al.* (1965, p.607–615) in a study of depressed patients with and without hypochondriacal symptoms, found that their hypochondriacal group had a 'significantly greater number of conspicuous environmental events coincident with the onset of the present illness' (1965, p.609). They cited illnesses in the family, death of a neighbour, emigration of a son, domestic conflicts and occupational stresses. In considering the aetiology of hypochondriacal symptoms, Kreitman and his collaborators found a few patients for whom they considered that the statement 'I am ill' seemingly meant 'I am lonely.' For others, 'I am ill' might signify, in addition to other meanings, 'I am in some kind of distress, but have learned no language other than my body by which to convey this.' Kreitman and his collaborators put forward a hypothesis, which focused on the hypochondriacal patient's interpersonal relations, particularly as these are reflected in marriage. They say:

> Since a somatic symptom can often elicit attention and concern on the part of a spouse and could therefore be used as a neurotic control mechanism when a psychological symptom could not, we predicted that the somatizing patients would have poorer marital relationships than the controls. This hypothesis was supported by the data and seems worthy of further study; even though alternative explanations of our findings are possible. It was striking how often the patients would start to describe their spouses' personality with the phrase, 'he's good to me when I'm ill' (1965, p.613–614).

Redlich and Freedman (1966) in their textbook of psychiatry emphasize how somatic complaints generate responses from others. They speak of hypochondriacal symptoms as 'providing "entrance tickets" for persons who feel neglected to win attention from a physician or to relate to a hospital or clinic setting'. For all of the abnormal illness behaviours, it is most useful to view these, although multi-factorially determined, as due largely to a desire to elicit increased care from others. This is demonstrated nowhere more so than in the grotesque features of the Munchausen syndrome (Cramer *et al.* 1971, p.576). Other forms of abnormal illness behaviour such as psychogenic pain and the widely varied presentations of compensation neurosis all become intelligible in terms of an economical theoretical structure. In each case, a developmentally primitive desire for care is to be found as a major factor in both the genesis of the disorder and in its perpetuation.

Anorexia nervosa

This syndrome, with its highest prevalence in young women for whom close personal relationships are a source of difficulty, is commonly found in families where food and eating are much stressed items in life. The young woman adopts two powerful signals for others to become concerned: she declines food and she becomes conspicuously thin. Both of these signals usually evoke anxiety in parents and subsequently in doctors and nurses. As a consequence, there is much expression of solicitude, which serves to reinforce the symptoms. It is not surprising that the syndrome is almost invariably long lasting and is conspicuous in its failure to respond to most treatment procedures. The success claimed for behaviour modification techniques (Bachrach *et al*. 1965, Stunkard 1972) may conceivably be attributed to the patient acquiring less injurious ways of obtaining attachment.

Shoplifting

A single label again subsumes a number of distinct syndromes. The type of shoplifting proposed as a care-eliciting syndrome is that occurring usually in middle-aged, middle-class women. Gibbens *et al*. describe a typical example:

> She is a woman of 50 who, a year before, had a hysterectomy and has not felt well since. She has backaches, headaches, dizziness, insomnia and a persistent sense of depression. She sometimes gets up in the night to turn off the gas or to see that the door is locked. She has no serious financial difficulties but her husband and children take no notice of her and she feels that life in the future stretches out like a desert. She has been seeing her doctor regularly and receiving tranquilizers but she has not been to him for 3 months because she feels she is wasting his time (1971, p.615).

The act of shoplifting for such a woman is so out of keeping with her usual behaviour and her usual value system that one is hard pressed to understand its motivation. A commonly proposed interpretation is that the behaviour is symptomatic of a depressive illness. Whether or not there is an affective disorder, the type of shoplifting described here is a behaviour, which is so incongruous that it can only be seen to express the following, though usually unconsciously:

1.   'Because of you, my life is empty.'

2.   'I am driven to do something quite grotesque.'

3.   'This will make you see how desperate I am for you to change.'

In addition, it is possible that some of the behaviour is accounted for by a regressive desire to acquire some trivial object, and perhaps also to be humiliated; all this in the one act. For treatment, the care-eliciting paradigm is a promising key to correcting some of the deficiencies in such women's lives.

Multiple illegitimate pregnancies

Illegitimate pregnancy in teenage girls undoubtedly has complex determinants, but the most conspicuous feature in the outcome is an increase in the amount of care shown to the girl herself. The girl usually has a marked desire for attachment and one method of securing this is to allow intimate sexual activity, thereby retaining the boy in a close relationship. Hollender *et al.* (1969, 1970) noted that in addition to intercourse being commonly used by women to entice their partner to hold them, this same desire is sometimes a determinant of promiscuity. Where there is a conscious desire to become pregnant and to have a baby, a further motivation is grafted on. This arises from the mechanism of projection, in which the girl is saying: 'If I have a baby, it will be looked after in the very way that I would myself like to be.' Indeed, as Babikian and Goldman (1971) have emphasized, there is usually an increase in the caring behaviour shown toward such girls, who commonly have endured an emotionally impoverished social environment.

DISCUSSION

The list of care-eliciting syndromes is probably incomplete. Indeed there is a danger that the concept suffers from over-inclusiveness, since for most diseases care-giving is a legitimate accompaniment. It is for this reason that strict criteria should be observed in the recognition of the syndromes. Minimum requirements are as follows:

1.   The behaviour or symptom is initiated by the individual himself, or is considered by professionals to have unconscious factors initiating it. This item helps differentiate, for example, psychogenic precordial pain from the symptoms and signs of myocardial ischaemia.

2.   The behaviour or symptom is appetitive.

3.   The behaviour or symptom is disruptive either for the individual
      or for others, or for both.

The disruptive character of the behaviour requires closer examination. It is
likely that the progression from normal to abnormal care-eliciting is dimensional rather than categorical, being a function of its degree of disruptiveness,
quite apart from its success in eliciting care. Parasuicide is an example of a
behaviour that, although often successful in evoking care, is markedly disruptive both for the individual and for others. By contrast, an isolated episode of a
wife weeping before her inattentive husband is in no way dissonant with the
behavioural norms of western societies. It seems reasonable, therefore, to define
as abnormal or deviant those care-eliciting behaviours, which exceed the limits
of tolerance either of the individual him/herself or of his/her society. It is clear
that not all deviant care-eliciting comes to the attention of professionals such as
doctors or police. Indeed, distressing patterns of care-eliciting are responsible
for much of the anxiety and hostility which are successfully, although painfully,
contained within families.

SEXUAL DIMORPHISM IN CARE-ELICITING BEHAVIOR

One of the most stable and recurrent findings in psychiatric epidemiology is
that females carry higher rates for neurotic disorder, commonly by a factor of
2:1 (Hagnell 1966, Lin and Standley 1962, Reid 1960, Shepherd and Cooper
1964, Srole et al. 1962, Taylor et al. 1964). This finding holds in most cultures
studied to date. Most of the care-eliciting syndromes have this same differential
in their sex incidence including those formally considered outside the neurotic
group, such as parasuicide and shoplifting. In considering normal
care-eliciting, it is important to bear in mind that the trait of dependency, particularly when marked, is more commonly observed in women in most cultures.
In the clinical situation, psychiatrists are more likely to recognize excessive
dependence in women than in men, whether or not one of the care-eliciting
syndromes is present. This recurrent sex difference may possibly be linked
ontogenetically with the observation that female infants separated from their
mothers tend to respond initially with an increase in attachment behaviour,
whereas boys tend to protest through aggression (Bowlby 1973). One tentative
conclusion to be drawn from these observations is that care-eliciting behaviour
may be more common in females throughout life. If this can be confirmed, it
would remain to be demonstrated that this is innate or biologically determined
in females, cultural factors accounting for very little of the difference. Two
observations are crucial in the investigation of this issue, the quantitative assess-

ment of care-eliciting behaviour in adult males and females, firstly in infrahuman primates and secondly in paleolithic or primitive hunting and gathering societies. It is only in the latter that one is likely to find those patterns of care-eliciting which were present in early man. If females in both groups are found to exceed males in this behaviour, it could go a long way toward establishing a biological basis for the greater attachment needs of females. Anthropological information of this type is not at present available for primitive societies, although in chimpanzees, Van Lawick-Goodall (1968) describes high status adult males rather than females being the recipients of most grooming. This, however, is an expression of the consequences of the dominance hierarchy; it tells us about the grooming received, not the grooming sought. Furthermore, as was discussed above, female chimpanzees have oestrus as a period when mating is assured whereas human females may have to rely on well-developed attachment behaviour to ensure the presence of a mate. Speculatively, this may be the key to the developmental origins of an important behavioural characteristic of women.

AMBIVALENCE OF RESPONSES

The care-eliciting syndromes share one other property; they tend to evoke ambivalent responses in others, particularly health professionals. This is most clearly seen in the attitudes of hospital staff to cases of parasuicide or abnormal illness behaviour. Liberman and Raskin (1971) correctly observed that neurotic depression can cause annoyance in others, as is commonly observed in the behaviour of many doctors toward patients with such symptoms. According to Parsons (1951), adoption of the sick role is permissible only when the disability is considered genuine and when the individual cooperates in efforts to return him to health. To assume the sick role in the absence of demonstrable or understandable disability is an infringement of the code relating to illness behaviour, a code that is held especially strongly by professionals designated as health workers. The inverse of this social structure relating to illness was very clearly pointed out in *Erewhon* by Samuel Butler (1872), where to be ill was to be punished and to be antisocial or dishonest was to be accorded sympathy and help.

Finally, it would go some way toward confirming the existence of the care-eliciting syndromes if it could be demonstrated that in persons suffering from any one of the disorders, there was an increased lifetime expectancy of developing one or more of the other syndromes. That is, in a group of persons who have carried out at least one act of parasuicide, is there an increased incidence, either previously or subsequently, of disorders such as neurotic depression, conversion hysteria, or abnormal illness behaviour? Such a question is eminently suitable for clinical investigation.

In conclusion, the concept of the care-eliciting syndromes, derived from the diverse fields of ethology, developmental psychology and clinical observation contributes toward a better understanding of the clinical aspects of this major category of behaviour.

NOTE

1   Foundation Professor of Psychiatry, University of Tasmania, Royal Hobart Hospital, Hobart, Australia 7000.

In developing the ideas expressed in this paper, the author is grateful to the following: Dr. John Bowlby, for much encouragement and useful criticism; Professor Derek Freeman, who initiated his interest in the subject; and Professor Robert Hinde.

The author acknowledges the following for their permission to use quotations: The Hogarth Press Ltd., and Basic Books. Inc. for the quotation by Dr. John Bowlby; Professor T. C. N. Gibbens, Drs. C. Palmer and J. Prince, the Editor and the British Medical Journal: Drs. N. Kreitman. P. Sainsbury, K. Pearce, and W. R. Costain, the Editor and the British Journal of Psychiatry.

REFERENCES

Babikian, H.M. and Goldman, A. (1971) A study in teenage pregnancy. *American Journal of Psychiatry*, 128, 755–760.

Bachrach, A.J., Erwin, W.J. and Mohr, J.P. (1965) 'The control of eating in an anorexic by operant conditioning techniques.' In L.P. Ullman and L. Ivrasner, eds. *Case Studies in Behaviour Modification.* New York: Holt, Rinehart and Winston.

Bowlby, J. (1969) *Attachment and Loss: Attachment, vol.1.* London: Hogarth Press.

Bowlby, J. (1973) *Attachment and Loss: Separation, vol.2.* London: Hogarth Press.

Butler, S. (1872) *Erewhon.* London: Trubner & Co.

Cramer, B., Gershberg, M.R. and Stern, M. (1971) Munchausen syndrome: Its relationship to malingering, hysteria and physician–patient relationship. *Archives of General Psychiatry*, 24, 573–578.

De Vore, I. (1963) 'Mother–infant relations in free-ranging baboons.' In H.L. Rheingold, ed. *Maternal Behaviour in Mammals.* New York: John Wiley.

Doi, L.T. (1969) 'Japanese psychology, dependency need, and mental health.' In J. Caudill and T. Lin, eds. *Mental Health Research in Asia and the Pacific.* Hawaii: East-West Center, University of Hawaii Press.

Eibl-Eibesfeldt, I. (1971) *Love and Hate: The Natural History of Behaviour Patterns.* New York: Holt, Rinehart and Winston.

Freud, S. (1946) *The Complete Psychological Works.* London: Hogarth Press.

Gibbens, T.C.N., Palmer, C. and Prince, J. (1971) Mental health aspects of shoplifting. *British Medical Journal*, 3, 612–615.

Guze, S.B. (1907) The diagnosis of hysteria: What are we trying to do? *American Journal of Psychiatry*, 124, 491–498.

Hagnell, O. (1966) *A Prospective Study of the Incidence of Mental Disorder.* Stockholm: Scandinavian University Books.

Hamburg, D. (1968) Evolution of emotional responses: Evidence from recent research on nonhuman primates. *Science and Psychoanalysis*, 12, 39–54.

Hamburg, D. (1971) Aggressive behaviour of chimpanzees and baboons in natural habitats. *Journal of Psychiatric Research*, 8, 385–398.

Harlow, H.F. (1960) Primary affectional patterns in primates. *American Journal of Orthopsychiatry*, 30, 676–684.

Harlow, M.K. and Harlow, H.F. (1966) Affection in primates. *Discovery*, 27, 11–17.

Hinde, R.A. (1970) 'Animal behaviour.' In *A Synthesis of Ethology and Comparative Psychology*, 2nd ed. Cambridge: Cambridge University Press.

Hinde, R.A. and Spencer-Booth, Y. (1971) Effects of brief separation from mother on rhesus monkeys. *Science*, 173, 111–118.

Hollender, M., Luborsky, L. and Harvey, R.B. (1970) Correlates of the desire to be held in women. *Journal of Psychosomatic Research*, 14, 387–390.

Hollender, M., Luborsky, L. and Scaramella, T.J. (1969) Body contact and sexual enticement. *Archives of General Psychiatry*, 20, 188–191.

Kendell, R.E. (1969) The continuum model of depressive illness. *Proceedings of the Royal Society of Medicine*, 62, 335–339.

Kiloh, L.G. and Garside, R.F. (1963) The independence of neurotic depression and endogenous depression. *British Journal of Psychiatry*, 109, 451–463.

Konner, M. J (1972) 'Aspects of the developmental ethology of a foraging people.' In N. Blurton-Jones, ed. *Ethological Studies of Child Behaviour.* Cambridge: Cambridge University Press.

Kraepelin, E. (1971) *Annual Reports, 1966–1971.* Munich: Max Planck Institute for Psychiatry. p.7.

Kreitman, N., Sainsbury, P., Pearce, K. and Coslain, W.R. (1965) Hypochondriasis and depression in outpatients at a general hospital. *British Journal of Psychiatry*, 111, 607–615.

Kreitman, N., Smith, P. and Tan, E.S. (1969) Attempted suicide in social networks. *British Journal of Preventative and Social Medicine*, 23, 110–123.

Kreitman, N., Smith, P. and Tan, E.S. (1970) Attempted suicide as language: An empirical study. *British Journal of Psychiatry*, 116, 465–473.

Lader, M. and Sartorius, N. (1968) Anxiety in patients with hysterical conversion symptoms. *Journal of Neurology, Neurosurgery and Psychiatry*, 31, 490–495.

Liberman, R.P. and Raskin, D.E. (1971) Depression: A behavioural formulation. *Archives of General Psychiatry*, 24, 515–523.

Lin, T. and Standley, C.C. (1962) *The Scope of Epidemiology in Psychiatry.* Geneva: World Health Organization Public Health Papers, No. 16.

Lorenz, K. (1966) *On Aggression.* London: Methuen.

Parens, H. and Saul, L.J. (1971) *Dependence in Man: A Psychoanalytic Study.* New York: International Universities Press.

Parsons, T. (1951) *The Social System.* Glencoe: The Free Press.

Paykel, E.S. (1971) Classification of depressed patients: A cluster-analysis-derived grouping. *British Journal of Psychiatry*, 118, 275–288.

Pilowsky, I. (1969) Abnormal illness behaviour. *British Journal of Medical Psychology*, 42, 347–351.

Redlich, F.C. and Freedman, D.X. (1966) *The Theory and Practice of Psychiatry*. New York: Basic Books.

Reid, D.D. (1960) *Epidemiological Methods in the Study of Menial Disorder*. Geneva: World Health Organization Public Health Papers, No. 2.

Rubinstein, R., Moses, R. and Litz, T. (1958) On attempted suicide. *Archives of Neurology and Psychiatry*, 79, 103–112.

Scott, J.P. (1969) The emotional basis of social behaviour. *Annals of the New York Academy of Sciences*, 160, 777–790.

Shepherd, M. and Cooper, B. (1964) Epidemiology and mental disorder: A review. *Journal of Neurology, Neurosurgery and Psychiatry*, 27, 277–290.

Slater, E. (1965) Diagnosis of 'hysteria'. *British Medical Journal*, 1, 1395–1399.

Sparks, J. (1967) 'Allogrooming in primates': A review. In D. Morris, ed. *Primate Ethology*. London: Weidenfeld and Nicolson.

Srole, L., Langner, T.S., Michael, S.T., Opler, M.K. and Rennie, T.A.C. (1962) *Mental Health in the Metropolis: The Midtown Manhattan Study*. New York: McGraw-Hill.

Stengel, E. (1964) *Suicide and Attempted Suicide*. England, Harmondsworth: Penguin.

Stunkard, A. (1972) New therapies for the eating disorders. *Archives of General Psychiatry*, 26, 391–398.

Surya, N.C. (1969) 'Ego structure in the Hindhu joint family: Some considerations.' In J. Caudill and T. Lin, eds. *Mental Health Research in Asia and the Pacific*. Hawaii: East-West Center, University of Hawaii Press, p.381.

Szasz, T.S. (1961) *The Myth of Mental Illness: Foundations of a Theory of Personal Conduct*. New York: Harper & Row.

Taylor, Lord and Chave, S. (1964) *Mental Health and Environment*. London: Longman's.

Tiger, L. (1969) *Men in Groups*. London: Nelson.

Van Lawick-Goodall, J. (1968) The behaviour of free-living chimpanzees in the Gombe stream reserve. *Animal Behaviour Monograms*, 1, (3).

. . . .

Points for reflective practice

- In considering your service-user group, what adversities have they faced in their past? How may these experiences shape or influence a service-user's perspective on the world and their relationships?

- Think about the attachment histories of the service users you work with. What was the experience for the service user of their family system; their parents, siblings and extended families? How does this help you understand their presentation?

- Think about an incident at work where a service user has acted in a way that engendered a response from the staff e.g. self-harming. How did you feel towards the service user? And towards the actions of other staff members during the incident? What could the service user be trying to communicate by their behaviour?

- What does 'care' mean to you? And to your service users?

. . . .

Part II

Clinical Implications

3

Hate in the Countertransference[*]

D.W. Winnicott
1947

. . . .

Editors' reflections

This classic paper is one of the first to acknowledge that therapists may experience ambivalent and indeed, hateful feelings towards service users during therapy. Also, due to the nature of their difficulties, there are a group of service users (the psychotics) who are more 'prone' to evoke these feelings. Countertransference subsequently becomes one of the central themes of the therapy. In recognising this, Winnicott makes a strong argument for personal therapy for those working with these individuals. By extension, we would take the view that all staff working in this field need to be offered, at a minimum, reflective space and supervision to explore negative feelings about service users openly and objectively.

. . . .

In this paper I wish to examine one aspect of the whole subject of ambivalence, namely, hate in the countertransference. I believe that the task of the analyst (call him a research analyst) who undertakes the analysis of a psychotic is seriously weighted by this phenomenon, and that analysis of psychotics becomes impossible unless the analyst's own hate is extremely well sorted-out and conscious. This is tantamount to saying that an analyst needs to be himself

[*] Originally published in D.W. Winnicott (1975) *Through Paediatrics to Psychoanalysis*. London: Hogarth Press, 194–203. Reprinted here by permission of Paterson Marsh Ltd on behalf of the Winnicott Trust.

analysed, but it also asserts that the analysis of a psychotic is irksome as compared with that of a neurotic, and inherently so.

Apart from psycho-analytic treatment, the management of a psychotic is bound to be irksome. From time to time I have made acutely critical remarks about the modern trends in psychiatry, with the too easy electric shocks and the too drastic leucotomies (Winnicott, 1947, 1949.) Because of these criticisms that I have expressed I would like to be foremost in recognition of the extreme difficulty inherent in the task of the psychiatrist, and of the mental nurse in particular. Insane patients must always be a heavy emotional burden on those who care for them. One can forgive those engaged in this work if they do awful things. This does not mean, however, that we have to accept whatever is done by psychiatrists and neuro-surgeons as sound according to principles of science.

Therefore although what follows is about psycho-analysis, it really has value to the psychiatrist, even to one whose work does not in any way take him into the analytic type of relationship to patients. To help the general psychiatrist the psycho-analyst must not only study for him the primitive stages of the emotional development of the ill individual, but also must study the nature of the emotional burden which the psychiatrist bears in doing his work. What we as analysts call the countertransference needs to be understood by the psychiatrist too. However much he loves his patients he cannot avoid hating them and fearing them, and the better he knows this the less will hate and fear be the motives determining what he does to his patients.

One could classify countertransference phenomena thus:

1. Abnormality in countertransference feelings and set relationships and identifications that are under repression in the analyst. The comment on this is that the analyst needs more analysis and we believe this is less of an issue among psycho-analysts than among psychotherapists in general.

2. The identifications and tendencies belonging to an analyst's personal experiences and personal development which provide the positive setting for his analytic work and make his work different in quality from that of any other analyst.

3. From these two I distinguish the truly objective countertransference, or if this is difficult, the analyst's love and hate in reaction to the actual personality and behaviour of the patient, based on objective observation.

I suggest that if an analyst is to analyse psychotics or antisocials he must be able to be so thoroughly aware of the countertransference that he can sort out and study his *objective* reactions to the patient. These will include hate. Countertransference phenomena will at times be the important things in the analysis.

I wish to suggest that the patient can only appreciate in the analyst what he himself is capable of feeling. In the matter of motive: the *obsessional* will tend to be thinking of the analyst as doing his work in a futile obsessional way. A *hypomanic* patient who is incapable of being depressed, except in a severe mood swing, and in whose emotional development the depressive position has not been securely won, who cannot feel guilt in a deep way, or a sense of concern or responsibility, is unable to see the analyst's work as an attempt on the part of the analyst to make reparation in respect of his own (the analyst's) guilt feelings. A *neurotic* patient tends to see the analyst as ambivalent towards the patient, and to expect the analyst to show a splitting of love and hate; this patient, when in luck, gets the love, because someone else is getting the analyst's hate. Would it not follow that if a *psychotic* is in a 'coincident love–hate' state of feeling he experiences a deep conviction that the analyst is also only capable of the same crude and dangerous state of coincident love–hate relationship? Should the analyst show love, he will surely at the same moment kill the patient.

This coincidence of love and hate is something that characteristically recurs in the analysis of psychotics, giving rise to problems of management which can easily take the analyst beyond his resources. This coincidence of love and hate to which I am referring is something distinct from the aggressive component complicating the primitive love impulse, and implies that, in the history of the patient, there was an environmental failure at the time of the first object-finding instinctual impulses. If the analyst is going to have crude feelings imputed to him he is best forewarned and so forearmed, for he must tolerate being placed in that position. Above all he must not deny hate that really exists in himself. Hate *that is justified* in the present setting has to be sorted out and kept in storage and available for eventual interpretation. If we are to become able to be the analysts of psychotic patients we must have reached down to very primitive things in ourselves, and this is but another example of the fact that the answer to many obscure problems of psycho-analytic practice lies in further analysis of the analyst. (Psycho-analytic research is perhaps always to some extent an attempt on the part of an analyst to carry the work of his own analysis further than the point to which his own analyst could get him.)

A main task of the analyst of any patient is to maintain objectivity in regard to all that the patient brings, and a special case of this is the analyst's need to be able to hate the patient objectively. Are there not many situations in our ordinary analytic work in which the analyst's hate is justified? A patient of mine, a very bad obsessional, was almost loathsome to me for some years. I felt bad about this until the analysis turned a corner and the patient became lovable, and then I realized that his unlikeableness had been an active symptom, unconsciously determined. It was indeed a wonderful day for me (much later on) when I could actually tell the patient that I and his friends had felt repelled by him, but that he had been too ill for us to let him know. This was also an important day for him, a tremendous advance in his adjustment to reality. In the ordinary analysis the analyst has no difficulty with the management of his own hate. This hate remains latent. The main thing, of course, is that through his own analysis he has become free from vast reservoirs of unconscious hate belonging to the past and to inner conflicts. There are other reasons why hate remains unexpressed and even unfelt as such:

> Analysis is my chosen job, the way I feel I will best deal with my own guilt, the way I can express myself in a constructive way.

> I get paid, or I am in training to gain a place in society by psychoanalytic work.

> I am discovering things.

> I get immediate rewards through identification with the patient, who is making progress, and I can see still greater rewards some way ahead, after the end of the treatment.

> Moreover, as an analyst I have ways of expressing hate. Hate is expressed by the existence of the end of the 'hour'.

I think this is true even when there is no difficulty whatever, and when the patient is pleased to go. In many analyses these things can be taken for granted, so that they are scarcely mentioned, and the analytic work is done through verbal interpretation of the patient's emerging unconscious transference. The analyst takes over the role of one or other of the helpful figures of the patient's childhood. He cashes in on the success of those who did the dirty work when the patient was an infant.

These things are part of the description of ordinary psycho-analytic work, which is mostly concerned with patients whose symptoms have a neurotic quality. In the analysis of psychotics, however, quite a different type and degree of strain is taken by the analyst, and it is precisely this different strain that I am trying to describe.

Recently for a period of a few days I found I was doing bad work. I made mistakes in respect of each one of my patients. The difficulty was in myself and it was partly personal but chiefly associated with a climax that I had reached in my relation to one particular psychotic (research) patient. The difficulty cleared up when I had what is sometimes called a 'healing' dream. (Incidentally I would add that during my analysis and in the years since the end of my analysis I have had a long series of these healing dreams which, although in many cases unpleasant, have each one of them marked my arrival at a new stage in emotional development.)

On this particular occasion I was aware of the meaning of the dream as I woke or even before I woke. The dream had two phases. In the first I was in the 'gods' in a theatre and looking down on the people a long way below in the stalls. I felt severe anxiety as if I might lose a limb. This was associated with the feeling I have had at the top of the Eiffel Tower that if I put my hand over the edge it would fall off on to the ground below. This would be ordinary castration anxiety.

In the next phase of the dream I was aware that the people in the stalls were watching a play and I was now related through them to what was going on on the stage. A new kind of anxiety now developed. What I knew was that I had no right side of my body at all. This was not a castration dream. It was a sense of not having that part of the body.

As I woke I was aware of having understood at a very deep level what was my difficulty at that particular time. The first part of the dream represented the ordinary anxieties that might develop in respect of unconscious fantasies of my neurotic patients. I would be in danger of losing my hand or my fingers if these patients should become interested in them. With this kind of anxiety I was familiar, and it was comparatively tolerable.

The second part of the dream, however, referred to my relation to the psychotic patient. This patient was requiring of me that I should have no relation to her body at all, not even an imaginative one; there was no body that she recognized as hers and if she existed at all she could only feel herself to be a mind. Any reference to her body produced paranoid anxieties, because to claim that she had a body was to persecute her. What she needed of me was that I should have only a mind speaking to her mind. At the culmination of my difficulties on the evening before the dream I had become irritated and had said that what she was needing of me was little better than hair-splitting. This had had a disastrous effect and it took many weeks for the analysis to recover from my lapse. The essential thing, however, was that I should understand my own anxiety and this was represented in the dream by the absence of the right side of my body when I tried to get into relation to the play that the people in the stalls were watching. This right side of my body was the side related to this particular patient and was therefore affected by her need to deny absolutely even an imaginative relationship of our bodies. This denial was producing in me this psychotic type of anxiety, much less tolerable than ordinary castration anxiety. Whatever other interpretations might be made in respect of this dream the result of my having dreamed it and remembered it was that I was able to take up this analysis again and even to heal the harm done to it by my irritability which had its origin in a reactive anxiety of a quality that was appropriate to my contact with a patient with no body.

The analyst must be prepared to bear strain without expecting the patient to know anything about what he is doing, perhaps over a long period of time. To do this he must be easily aware of his own fear and hate. He is in the position of the mother of an infant unborn or newly born. Eventually, he ought to be able to tell his patient what he has been through on the patient's behalf, but an analysis may never get as far as this. There may be too little good experience in the patient's past to work on. What if there be no satisfactory relationship of early infancy for the analyst to exploit in the transference?

There is a vast difference between those patients who have had satisfactory early experiences which can be discovered in the transference, and those whose very early experiences have been so deficient or distorted that the analyst has to be the first in the patient's life to supply certain environmental essentials. In the treatment of a patient of the latter kind all sorts of things in analytic technique become vitally important, things that can be taken for granted in the treatment of patients of the former type.

I asked a colleague whether he does analysis in the dark, and he said: 'Why, no! Surely our job is to provide an ordinary environment: and the dark would be extraordinary'. He was surprised at my question. He was orientated towards analysis of neurotics. But this provision and maintenance of an ordinary environment can be in itself a vitally important thing in the analysis of a psychotic, in fact it can be, at times, even more important than the verbal interpretations which also have to be given. For the neurotic the couch and warmth and comfort can be *symbolical* of the mother's love; for the psychotic it would be more true to say that these things *are* the analyst's physical expression of love. The couch *is* the analyst's lap or womb, and the warmth *is* the live warmth of the analyst's body. And so on.

There is, I hope, a progression in my statement of my subject. The analyst's hate is ordinarily latent and is easily kept so. In analysis of psychotics the analyst is under greater strain to keep his hate latent, and he can only do this by being thoroughly aware of it. I want to add that in certain stages of certain analyses the analyst's hate is actually sought by the patient, and what is then needed is hate that is objective. If the patient seeks objective or justified hate he must be able to reach it, else he cannot feel he can reach objective love.

It is perhaps relevant here to cite the case of the child of the broken home, or the child without parents. Such a child spends his time unconsciously looking for his parents. It is notoriously inadequate to take such a child into one's home and to love him. What happens is that after a while a child so adopted gains hope, and then he starts to test out the environment he has found, and to seek proof of his guardians' ability to hate objectively. It seems that he can believe in being loved only after reaching being hated.

During the Second World War a boy of nine came to a hostel for evacuated children, sent from London not because of bombs but because of truancy. I hoped to give him some treatment during his stay in the hostel, but his symptom won and he ran away as he had always done from everywhere since the age of six when he first ran away from home. However, I had established contact with him in one interview in which I could see and interpret through a drawing of his that in running away he was unconsciously saving the inside of his home and preserving his mother from assault, as well as trying to get away from his own inner world, which was full of persecutors.

I was not very surprised when he turned up in the police station very near my home. This was one of the few police stations that did not know him intimately. My wife very generously took him in and kept him for three months, three months of hell. He was the most lovable and most maddening of children, often stark staring mad. But fortunately we knew what to expect. We dealt with the first phase by giving him complete freedom and a shilling whenever he went out. He had only to ring up and we fetched him from whatever police station had taken charge of him.

Soon the expected change-over occurred, the truancy symptom turned round, and the boy started dramatizing the assault on the inside. It was really a whole-time job for the two of us together, and when I was out the worst episodes took place.

Interpretation had to be made at any minute of day or night, and often the only solution in a crisis was to make the correct interpretation, as if the boy were in analysis. It was the correct interpretation that he valued above everything.

The important thing for the purpose of this paper is the way in which the evolution of the boy's personality engendered hate in me, and what I did about it. Did I hit him? The answer is no, I never hit. But I should have had to have done so if I had not known all about my hate and if I had not let him know about it too. At crises I would take him by bodily strength, without anger or blame, and put him outside the front door, whatever the weather or the time of day or night. There was a special bell he could ring, and he knew that if he rang it he would be readmitted and no word said about the past. He used this bell as soon as he had recovered from his maniacal attack.

The important thing is that each time, just as I put him outside the door, I told him something; I said that what had happened had made me hate him. This was easy because it was so true. I think these words were important from the point of view of his progress, but they were mainly important in enabling me to tolerate the situation without letting out, without losing my temper and without every now and again murdering him. This boy's full story cannot be told here. He went to an Approved School. His deeply rooted relation to us has remained one of the few stable things in his life. This episode from ordinary life can be used to illustrate the general topic of hate justified in the present; this is to be distinguished from hate that is only justified in another setting but which is tapped by some action of a patient.

Out of all the complexity of the problem of hate and its roots I want to rescue one thing, because I believe it has an importance for the analyst of psychotic patients. I suggest that the mother hates the baby before the baby hates the mother, and before the baby can know his mother hates him.

Before developing this theme I want to refer to Freud. In *Instincts and their Vicissitudes* (1915), where he says so much that is original and illuminating about hate, Freud says: 'We might at a pinch say of an instinct that it "loves" the objects after which it strives for purposes of satisfaction, but to say that it "hates" an object strikes us as odd, so we become aware that the attitudes of love and hate cannot be said to characterize the relation of instincts to their objects, but are reserved for the relations of the ego as a whole to objects...' This I feel is true and important. Does this not mean that the personality must be integrated before an infant can be said to hate? However early integration may be achieved—perhaps integration occurs earliest at the height of excitement or rage—there is a theoretical earlier stage in which whatever the infant does that hurts is not done in hate. I have used the term 'ruthless love' in describing this stage. Is this acceptable? As the infant becomes able to feel to be a whole person, so does the word hate develop meaning as a description of a certain group of his feelings.

The mother, however, hates her infant from the word go. I believe Freud thought it possible that a mother may in certain circumstances have only love for her boy baby; but we may doubt this. We know about a mother's love and we appreciate its reality and power. Let me give some of the reasons why a mother hates her baby, even a boy:

The baby is not her own (mental) conception.

The baby is not the one of childhood play, father's child, brother's child, etc.

The baby is not magically produced.

The baby is a danger to her body in pregnancy and at birth.

The baby is an interference with her private life, a challenge to preoccupation.

To a greater or lesser extent a mother feels that her own mother demands a baby, so that her baby is produced to placate her mother.

The baby hurts her nipples even by suckling, which is at first a chewing activity.

He is ruthless, treats her as scum, an unpaid servant, a slave.

She has to love him, excretions and all, at any rate at the beginning, till he has doubts about himself.

He tries to hurt her, periodically bites her, all in love.

He shows disillusionment about her.

His excited love is cupboard love, so that having got what he wants he throws her away like orange peel.

The baby at first must dominate, he must be protected from coincidences, life must unfold at the baby's rate and all this needs his mother's continuous and detailed study. For instance, she must not be anxious when holding him, etc.

At first he does not know at all what she does or what she sacrifices for him. Especially he cannot allow for her hate.

He is suspicious, refuses her good food, and makes her doubt herself, but eats well with his aunt.

After an awful morning with him she goes out, and he smiles at a stranger, who says: 'Isn't he sweet?'

If she fails him at the start she knows he will pay her out for ever.

He excites her but frustrates—she mustn't eat him or trade in sex with him.

I think that in the analysis of psychotics, and in the ultimate stages of the analysis, even of a normal person, the analyst must find himself in a position comparable to that of the mother of a new-born baby. When deeply regressed the patient cannot identify with the analyst or appreciate his point of view any more than the foetus or newly born infant can sympathize with the mother. A mother has to be able to tolerate hating her baby without doing anything about it. She cannot express it to him. If, for fear of what she may do, she cannot hate appropriately when hurt by her child she must fall back on masochism, and I think it is this that gives rise to the false theory of a natural masochism in women. The most remarkable thing about a mother is her ability to be hurt so much by her baby and to hate so much without paying the child out, and her ability to wait for rewards that may or may not come at a later date. Perhaps she is helped by some of the nursery rhymes she sings, which her baby enjoys but fortunately does not understand?

> Rockabye Baby, on the tree top,
> When the wind blows the cradle will rock,
> When the bough breaks the cradle will fall,
> Down will come baby, cradle and all.

I think of a mother (or father) playing with a small infant; the infant enjoying the play and not knowing that the parent is expressing hate in the words, perhaps in terms of birth symbolism. This is not a sentimental rhyme. Sentimentality is useless for parents, as it contains a denial of hate, and sentimentality in a mother is no good at all from the infant's point of view. It seems to me doubtful whether a human child as he develops is capable of tolerating the full extent of his own hate in a sentimental environment. He needs hate to hate. If this is true, a psychotic patient in analysis cannot be expected to tolerate his hate of the analyst unless the analyst can hate him.

If all this is accepted there remains for discussion the question of the interpretation of the analyst's hate to the patient. This is obviously a matter fraught with danger, and it needs the most careful timing. But I believe an analysis is incomplete if even towards the end it has not been possible for the analyst to tell the patient what he, the analyst, did unbeknown for the patient whilst he was ill, in the early stages. Until this interpretation is made the patient is kept to some extent in the position of infant—one who cannot understand what he owes to his mother.

An analyst has to display all the patience and tolerance and reliability of a mother devoted to her infant; has to recognize the patient's wishes as needs;

has to put aside other interests in order to be available and to be punctual and objective; and has to seem to want to give what is really only given because of the patient's needs. There may be a long initial period in which the analyst's point of view cannot be appreciated (even unconsciously) by the patient. Acknowledgement cannot be expected because, at the primitive root of the patient that is being looked for, there is no capacity for identification with the analyst; and certainly the patient cannot see that the analyst's hate is often engendered by the very things the patient does in his crude way of loving.

In the analysis (research analysis) or in ordinary management of the more psychotic type of patient, a great strain is put on the analyst (psychiatrist, mental nurse) and it is important to study the ways in which anxiety of psychotic quality and also hate are produced in those who work with severely ill psychiatric patients. Only in this way can there be any hope of the avoidance of therapy that is adapted to the needs of the therapist rather than to the needs of the patient.

4

Taking Care of the Hateful Patient*

James E. Groves
1978

. . . .

Editors' reflections

This next American paper is written about physicians working with patients in general medical practice. It is interesting because it links the practice of general medicine with that of psychotherapy, psychiatry and forensic psychiatry; and so indicates that hateful feelings towards some service users are an inevitable part of clinical practice. Groves cites Winnicott's paper; and describes the phenomenon that is called by later authors, 'malignant alienation'. What this paper also raises is the extent to which the vulnerable are hated by those who care for them. Although we like to think of people being very caring and tender towards the vulnerable, in other mammalian groups, vulnerable and needy individuals are often excluded and rejected. The other possibility is that we feel hostile towards the vulnerable because they remind us of our own neediness. However construed, it seems that feelings of hate are to be expected in the care of some service users, and as Groves suggests, the sooner we get on and explore them, the better.

. . . .

Abstract

"Hateful patients" are not those with whom the physician has an occasional personality clash. As defined here, they are those whom most physicians dread. The insatiable dependency of "hateful patients" leads to behaviors that group them into four stereotypes: dependent clingers, entitled demanders, manipulative help-rejecters and self-destructive deniers.

The physician's negative reactions constitute important clinical data that should facilitate better understanding and more appropriate psychological management for each. Clingers evoke aversion; their care requires limits on expectations for an intense doctor–patient relationship. Demanders evoke a wish to counterattack; such patients need to have their feelings of total entitlement rechanneled into a partnership that acknowledges their entitlement—not to unrealistic demands but to good medical care. Help-rejecters evoke depression; "sharing" their pessimism diminishes their notion that losing the symptom implies losing the doctor. Self-destructive deniers evoke feelings of malice; their management requires the physician to lower Faustian expectations of delivering perfect care.

INTRODUCTION

Admitted or not, the fact remains that a few patients kindle aversion, fear, despair or even downright malice in their doctors. Emotional reactions to patients cannot simply be wished away, nor is it good medicine to pretend that they do not exist. Doctors cannot avoid occasional negative feelings toward the "obnoxious patient" (Martin, 1975) the whining "self-pitier" (Hackett, 1969) or the help-rejecting "crock" (Lipsitt, 1970). Like that of Faust, the doctor's ideal is to "know all, love all, heal all," (Maltsberger and Buie, 1974) but when this ideal of the perfect physician collides with the quotidian realities of caring for sick and troubled patients, a number of processes may ensue: there may be "helplessness in the helper" (Adler, 1972); there may be unconscious punishment of the patient (Hackett, 1969); there may be self-punishment by the doctor (Maltsberger and Buie 1974); there may be inappropriate confrontation of the patient (Adler and Buie, 1972); and there may be a desperate attempt to avoid or to extrude the patient from the care-giving system (Bibring, 1956; Groves, 1978).

A 51-year-old attorney specializing in medical negligence was enraged when his many complaints were ultimately diagnosed as multiple sclerosis. Known for his flashy wardrobe and courtroom pyrotechnics, he roamed from doctor to doctor, refusing to understand the nature of his illness and threatening to sue the previous "bastard" who had tried to help him. He was like Job (xiii:4), who raged, "ye are forgers of lies, ye are all physicians of no value." He adamantly refused treatment and demanded more and more tests and consultations. Eventually, his doctors did not return his calls for appointments and were frightened and depressed about him. How long this situation might have continued is not known, because at this point—to the relief of all concerned—he was stopped by an exacerbation of his demyelinating process that required hospitalization in a chronic-care facility.

This vignette illustrates a "hateful patient"—one whom most physicians would dread to treat. The present communication addresses "countertransference" feelings toward the patient, except for two situations that are thoroughly treated elsewhere: feelings toward the obviously suicidal patient (Maltsberger and Buie, 1974); and idiosyncratic bias reactions confined to a particular doctor with certain kinds of patients (Bibring, 1956; Hackett, 1969). The latter group of reactions is determined by specific psychologic processes (usually unconscious) in one doctor; in such a case, the remedy of transferring the patient may well be appropriate, since the idiosyncrasies of one physician are not highly likely to be those of another. Here, discussion will center on patients for whom most physicians would harbor negative feelings and for whom transfer is not usually helpful to the patient.

HATE IN THE LITERATURE OF MEDICINE

The medical student and the doctor find little help in the literature. Even Osler (1935) fails in this regard. Nowhere in his *Principles and Practice of Medicine* does he allude to personal feelings that the difficult patient may stir up; his other writings (Osler 1943 and 1951) are sermons, more inspirational than practical. Modern textbooks of medicine have a few pages on the doctor–patient relationship (Beeson and McDermott, 1975; Thorn *et al.*, 1977) but their most negative appellation for a patient is "exasperating," (Thorn *et al.*, 1977) and they generally suggest that the physician disown negative feelings in favor of integrity, truth, humor and compassion. Psychiatry too, with certain notable exceptions, (Bibring, 1956; Hackett, 1969; Lipsitt, 1970) has failed to help the rest of medicine with the feelings that patients stir up; even when feelings are addressed directly (Kolb, 1963) the advice tendered is most likely to be, transfer to a colleague who can stand the patient. This gap is particularly odd because psychiatry has been fascinated with the negative side of the doctor–patient relationship since the turn of the century.

"Countertransference" is the word that Freud coined to mean emotional reactions to a patient that are determined by the psychoanalyst's own unconscious conflict. Later on, "countertransference" assumed for some a broader meaning of unconscious and conscious unbidden and unwanted hostile and sexual feelings toward the patient—feelings that were seen to impede the treatment and to reflect poorly on the analyst. Although Freud himself was rather candid about his own countertransference reactions his scientific attitude about it was often difficult for his early followers to emulate.

In 1949 the prestigious *International Journal of Psycho-Analysis* published a paper written by a pediatrician and psychoanalyst named D. W. Winnicott and entitled "Hate in the Countertransference" (Winnicott, 1949). In it he acknowledged outright hatred for some patients in certain circumstances. This hatred—and even the murderous wishes associated with it—he compared with the occasional inevitable dislike of the mother for her demanding infant. He noted apparent innocence of nursery rhymes and lullabys betrays such hatred mixed with maternal love ("Down will come baby/Cradle and all"). The publication of "Hate in the Countertransference" was a benchmark in the study of such feelings; subsequently, papers about countertransference were less defensive. Such feelings have gradually come to be regarded not only as a painful visitation but also as a necessary clue guiding the psychiatrist's conceptualization and technique. Likewise, the study of countertransference phenomena can guide other physicians, especially in the management of four classes of patients: dependent *clingers*; entitled *demanders*; manipulative *help-rejecters*; and self-destructive *deniers*. At times, a single patient may epitomize more than one of these classes. The following portraits are stereotypes.

DEPENDENT CLINGERS

Clingers escalate from mild and appropriate requests for reassurance to repeated, perfervid, incarcerating cries for explanation, affection, analgesics, sedatives and all forms of attention imaginable. They are naive about their effect on the physician, and they are overt in their neediness. They may have no discernible medical illness, or they may have severe chronic or life-threatening disorders; but whatever their medical problems, what is common to them as a group is their self-perception of bottomless need and their perception of the physician as inexhaustible. Such dependency may eventually lead to a sense of weary aversion toward the patient. When the doctor's stamina is exhausted, a referral for psychiatric examination may be adamantly put forth in frustrated tones that the patient (correctly) interprets as rejection. Psychiatric referrals made in this context are destined to fail utterly.

> A 23-year-old "exotic dancer" of no little beauty consulted a resident in medicine because of fatigue. This male resident was eventually able to make the diagnosis of lupus. He took care in explaining the mild nature of her particular course. She responded intelligently with questions pertinent to prognosis and eventually asked him whether he would follow her, long-term, for this chronic illness. Flattered and touched, he vowed to do so. Later that day she telephoned briefly to thank him.
>
> During the next week she visited with a question about her medication. In the following week she called twice, once professing great fear that she would die and another time to thank him again. As weeks passed, her calls and visits became more frequent, and her thanks dwindled to nothing. He began to dread her calls.
>
> By the end of two months she was calling him daily, in the office and at home. What had begun as a minuet ultimately became a fandango. He changed programs; she soon was involved in a similar situation with another resident in the same clinic.

Early signs of the clinger are the patient's genuine gratitude but to an extreme degree, and the doctor's feelings of power and specialness to the patient, an emotion not unlike puppy love. Later on, the doctor and the patient have different feelings toward each other. The doctor becomes the inexhaustible mother; the patient becomes the unplanned, unwanted, unlovable child. Early identification of this situation is helpful, but its corrective may be applied—if done skillfully—at any point short of a complete blowup. The clinger must be told as early in the relationship as possible, and as tactfully and firmly as possible, that the physician has not only human limits to knowledge and skill but also limitations to time and stamina. Written follow-up appointments are placed in the patient's hand, the doctor says, "so long," and never, "good-bye," and the patient is firmly reminded not to call except during office hours or in an emergency. This approach is not cruelty or rejection. It is in the best interest of patient care to protect the patient from promises that cannot be kept and from illusions that are bound to shatter.

ENTITLED DEMANDERS

Demanders resemble clingers in the profundity of their neediness, but they differ in that—rather than flattery and unconscious seduction—they use intimidation, devaluation and guilt-induction to place the doctor in the role of the inexhaustible, supply depot. They appear less naive about their effect on the physician than clingers and buttress their hold on the doctor by threatening punishment. The patient may try to control the physician by withholding payment or threatening litigation. The patient is unaware of the deep dependency that underlies these attacks on the doctor. The physician, in turn, does not recognize that the hostility is born of terror of abandonment. Moreover, such patients often exude a repulsive sense of innate deservedness as if they were far superior to the physician. This attitude is to shield them from awareness that the physician seems to have power over life and death. Obviously, this sense of innate and magical entitlement to everything that is wanted is depressing (and therefore often enraging) to the busy physician, who may have had to surrender many streams of omnipotence and omniscience over the years of training. The physician becomes fearful about his reputation, enraged that the patient is not co-operative and grateful; and—eventually—secretly self-blaming as if the patient's devaluating demands are realistic. But this very "entitlement," repulsive as it may be, is resorted to by the patient in an effort to preserve the integrity of the self in a world that seems hostile or, during an illness, that seems terrifying. "Entitlement" serves for some persons the functions that faith and hope serve in better adjusted ones. The usual impulse toward entitlement is a wish to point out suddenly and devastatingly that the patient has earned little, medically or in larger society, and deserves little. But this course would be an assault on the very psychological foundations that support such a patient. Entitlement is such a patient's religion and should not be blasphemed.

Because the lawyer with multiple sclerosis in the first vignette was entitled, he was vulnerable to counterattack. But because he had so much actual power to harm his caregivers, counterattack did not in fact occur. Because his terror and entitlement were concealed beneath the trappings of real achievement, neither was his bombast recognized for what it was—a pathetic sham. Thus it was not addressed in service of the patient's best interest. The physician should never gainsay the patient's entitlement. The most helpful therapeutic strategy with the entitled demander is to support the entitlement but to rechannel it in the direction of the indicated regimen. His doctor might have said,

> I know you're mad about this and mad at the other doctors. You have reason to be mad. You have an illness that makes some people give up, and you're fighting it. But you're fighting your doctors too. You say you're

entitled to repeated tests, damages for suffering and all that. And you are entitled—entitled to the very best medical care we can give you. But we can't give you the good treatment you deserve unless you help. You deserve a chance to control this disease; you deserve all the allies you can get. You'll get the help you deserve if you'll stop misdirecting your anger to the very people who are trying to help you get what you deserve—good medical care.

Such an approach acknowledges the patient's entitlement—not to have unreasonable demands met or to bully others but to what is realistically good care. The physician must be aware of the litigiousness of such patients and may to a certain extent practice "defensive medicine," but need not be bullied or actually defensive. The doctor also should beware of getting entangled in complicated logical (or illogical) debates with the patient. Rather, there should be tireless repetition of the theme of acceptance that the patient deserves first-rate medical care.

MANIPULATIVE HELP-REJECTERS

Help-rejecters, or "crocks," (Lipsitt, 1970) are familiar to every practicing physician. Like clingers and demanders, they appear to have a quenchless need for emotional supplies. Unlike clingers, they are not seductive and grateful; unlike demanders they are not overtly hostile. They actually seem the opposite of entitled; they appear to feel that no regimen will help. Appearing almost smugly satisfied, they return again and again to the office or clinic to report that, once again, the regimen did not work. Their pessimism and tenacious nay-saying appear to increase in direct proportion to the physician's efforts and enthusiasm. When one of their symptoms is relieved, another mysteriously appears in its place. Apparently, what is sought is not relief of symptoms. What is sought is an undivorcible marriage with an inexhaustible caregiver. Such patients seem to use their symptoms as an admission ticket to a relationship that cannot be sundered so long as symptoms exist. Thus, they are often accused of "masochism" and are said to be reaping unjustified "secondary gain." Such patients, frequently deny being depressed and typically refuse referral to a psychiatrist. Lipsitt (1970) records the case of one such patient who had 10 operations in 12 years, multiple visits to a dozen clinics and a chart that was four volumes long. "Only once was the term depression mentioned in…her record and that appeared in…1956," some 13 years after she had begun her hegira. Another patient whom he studied had 829 visits to 26 clinics in 36 years; she "said of herself, 'I have a *bissel of tsuri*'" (a smidgin of trouble).

These behaviors elicit first in the physician anxiety that a treatable illness has been overlooked, next irritation with the patient and, finally, depression and self-doubt in the doctor. But the depression originally is not in the doctor—it is usually in the patient. Although it is important to suspect depression in the help-rejecter, it is hazardous to imply that he or she is too dependent or immature to get better or that unconscious manipulation is going on. Such an approach simply precipitates a new round of doctor-shopping. Rather, it may be helpful to "share" the pessimism—to say that the treatment may not be entirely curative. Even if it is, regular follow-up visits (hence, at intervals determined by the doctor) are put forth as necessary for the maintenance of any modest gains. In this way, the patient's fear of losing the doctor may be partly allayed, and the patient may be able to follow the treatment plan without fear of engineering his or her own abandonment.

Pathologic dependency presents in one of its extremes as *manipulativeness*— an intense, covert, contradictory, self-defeating attempt to get needs met. It is the behavioral manifestation of a need by the patient to get close to but at the same time to maintain safe distance from sources of emotional support. (Occasional patients feel so empty that, paradoxically, to get needs met threatens them with engulfment; they are so famished that closeness may actually make them feel merged with someone else and therefore not really alive.) Such patients seem to have a deathly fear of that which they most crave (Groves, 1978).

A young woman in her twenties was hospitalized for control of Brittle diabetes mellitus. Cachectic and hateful, she appeared to drive people away. She had a long history of psychiatric hospitalizations, multiple suicide attempts, abysmal relationships and an implacable resistance to co-operating in the management of her illness. Yet she clung to hospitalization. On the day before discharge she simultaneously infected her intravenous lines with faeces and spiked a high temperature and threatened to sign out against medical advice. Raging and septic, she had to be physically restrained from leaving prematurely.

The remedy here is not to interpret the pathologic "solution" to the "need/fear dilemma," which is unconsciously being acted out by the patient. Such an action would be useless and harmful. Rather, limits on unrealistic expectations, limits on demanding hostility and—most of all—repeated appeals to entitlement are again invoked. The doctor, by a consistent, firm manner, conveys that the patient will not be allowed to become so close as to be engulfed nor so distant as to starve. Gentle, simple reasoning with this patient is better than complicated explanations.

To refer help-rejecters for psychiatric evaluation is never easy. If a psychiatric illness is thought to be present, one tactic for helping the patient accept psychiatric consultation is to schedule another appointment with the patient for a time after the consultation is to occur. In this way, the doctor can convey that the consultation is an adjunct to medical treatment, not abandonment.

SELF-DESTRUCTIVE DENIERS

Self-destructive deniers display unconsciously self-murderous behaviors, such as the continued drinking of a patient with esophageal varices and hepatic failure. This type of denial must be distinguished from other forms of denial, such as the "forgetting" of a brawny cardiac patient told not to shovel snow—a type of denial that evokes anxiety in the physician. Grossly self-destructive denial, on the other hand stirs up malice. To make this distinction, it is important first to recognize that some patients—called "major deniers" (Hackett and Cassem, 1970)—deny without any self-destructive intent. They prize their independence and deny infirmity and chafe bitterly under the restrictions that a medical regimen imposes. But their denial is probably adaptive because they appear to survive longer than nondeniers (Hackett and Cassem, 1970). The doctor working with a "major denier" should work cheerfully with the denial. Appeals to the patient's sense of sturdiness are harnessed to the necessary regimen. "Major deniers" tend to be likable and hard-working patients who respond to person-to-person medical advice delivered with a light touch and focused on maintenance of good health. Doomsaying, authoritarian approaches typically fail because the patient easily denies bad news.

The self-destructive denier is an entirely different story. Such patients are not independent and using the defense of denial in an attempt to survive. Rather they are at base profoundly dependent and have given up hope of ever having needs met. Such patients seem to glory in their own destruction. They appear to find their main pleasure in furiously defeating the physician's attempts to preserve their lives. They may represent a chronic form of suicidal behavior; often they let themselves die.

A 45-year-old alcoholic man was familiarly called "Old George" by members of the emergency-ward staff. They had seen him a hundred times over six years for visits ranging from acute gastrointestinal bleeds to a subdural hematoma (after a fall that he barely survived). It became a standing joke that the more carefully Old George was tended and the more thoroughly he was worked up, the more furiously he drank. He was released from his hospitalization for the subdural hematoma on Monday, stitched up for multiple lacerations on Tuesday, allowed to "sleep it off" in the back hall on Wednesday, casted for a fractured arm on Thursday and admitted with wildly bleeding esophageal varices on Friday. The staff worked frantically through the night, pumping in whole blood as fast as it would go, but at 4 a.m. the intern pronounced Old George dead, the junior resident muttered, "thank God," under his breath, and the senior resident said, "Amen," quite audibly.

What the physician can do to help self-destructive deniers is quite limited. The starting point for the care of such a patient is to recognize without shame or self-blame that they provoke in their caregivers the fervent wish that they would die and "get it over with." Many physicians, recognizing in themselves such a wish, recoil—by temperament and by training. When the doctor encounters the expertly self-destructive patient, he or she is caught between the ideal of rescuing the patient on one hand and the unwanted wish for the patient to die on the other. Depending on how mature the physician is about such hateful feelings, malice toward the patient will be either conscious and associated with little guilt or self-reproach (Maltsberger and Buie, 1974) or hidden and a cause of feelings of dread, self-blame, gratuitously heroic rescue efforts or a flat, bland, given-up and hopeless attitude. The optimal care of the chronically self-murderous patient entails a psychiatric consultation for the patient to ascertain whether treatable depression exists. If the patient refuses such a consultation (and most do) the primary physician may have to fight the impulse to abandon the patient. It is crucial to recognize the limitations that such patients pose for even the most ideal care givers and to work with diligence and compassion to preserve the denier as long as possible, just as one does with any other patient with a terminal illness.

DISCUSSION

The "hateful patient," then, is the patient who—by a variety of behaviors related to profound dependency—stimulates a series of negative feelings in most doctors. Dependent *clingers* evoke aversion. Entitled *demanders* evoke fear and then counterattack upon entitlement. Manipulative *help-rejecters* evoke guilt and feelings of inadequacy. Self-destructive *deniers* (unlike "major deniers," who generally stir up affection mingled with anxiety) evoke all these negative feelings, as well as malice and, at times, the secret wish that the patient will "die and get it over with."

Day in and day out, however, the physician routinely helps most patients establish better contact with reality, better adaptation to painful illnesses and better relations with families, friends and other care givers. What is it about the patient "everybody hates" that compromises these workaday skills? It is probably the additional burden of having to deny or disown the intense, hateful feelings kindled by the dependent, entitled, manipulative or self-destructive patient. What the behaviors of such patients teach over time is that it is not how one feels about them that is most important in their care. It is how one behaves toward them: the doctor who begins to feel aversion toward the patient should begin to think of setting limits on dependency. The doctor who begins to feel the impulse to counterattack should begin to think of rechanneling entitlement into expectations of realistically good medical care. The doctor who begins to feel depressed with the patient's smug help-rejecting should begin to think of "sharing pessimism" so that the patient's losing the symptom is not equated with losing the doctor. And the doctor who begins to wish that the patient would die should begin to grasp the possibility that the patient wishes to die.

Negative feelings about medical and surgical patients constitute important clinical data about the patient's psychology. When the patient creates in the doctor feelings that are disowned or denied, errors in diagnosis and treatment are more likely to occur. Disavowal of hateful feelings requires less effort than bearing them. But such disavowal wastes clinical data that may be helpful in treating the "hateful patient."

I am indebted to Drs. Ross J. Baldessarini and John D. Stoeckle for criticism of early versions of the manuscript and to Dr. Thomas P. Hackett for encouragement and suggestions throughout.

REFERENCES

Adler, G. (1972) Helplessness in the helpers. *British Journal of Medical Psychology*, 45, 315–326.

Adler, G. and Buie, D.H. (1972) The misuses of confrontation with borderline patients. *International Journal of Psychoanalytic Psychotherapy*, 1, 109–120.

Beeson, P.B. and McDermott, W. eds. (1975) *Cecil-Loeb Textbook of Medicine.* Philadelphia: WB Saunders.

Bibring, G.L. (1956) Psychiatry and medical practice in a general hospital. *New England Journal of Medicine*, 254, 366–372.

Groves, J.E. (1975) Management of the borderline patient on a medical or surgical ward: the psychiatric consultant's role. *International Journal of Psychiatry and Medicine*, 6, 337–348.

Groves, J.E. (1978) 'Violence and sociopathy in the general hospital: psychotic and borderline patients on medical and surgical wards.' In T.P. Hackett and N.H. Cassem, eds. *The MGH Handbook of Liaison Psychiatry.* St Louis: CV Mosby.

Hackett, T.P. (1969) Which patients turn you off? It's worth analyzing. *Medicine and Economics,* 46 (15), 94–99.

Hackett, T.P. and Cassem, N.H. (1970) *Psychological reactions to life-threatening illness, psychological aspects of stress.* Edited by H. Abram. Springfield, Illinois: CC Thomas. p.29–43.

Kolb, L.C. (1963) 'The psychoneuroses.' In P.B. Beeson and W. McDermott eds. (1963) *Cecil-Loeb Textbook of Medicine.* 11th ed. Philadelphia: WB Saunders. p.1709–1727.

Lipsitt, D.R. (1970) Medical and psychological characteristics of "crocks." *International Journal of Psychiatry and Medicine,* 1, 15–25.

Maltsberger, J.T. and Buie, D.H. (1974) Countertransference hate in the treatment of suicidal patients. *Archives of General Psychiatry,* 30, 625–633.

Martin, P.A. (1975) 'The obnoxious patient: tactics and techniques.' In P.L. Giovacchini, ed. *Psychoanalytic Therapy. Vol 2. Countertransference.* New York: Jason Aronson. p.196–204.

Osler, W. (1935) *Principles and Practice of Medicine.* 12th ed. Edited by T. McCrae. New York: Appleton-Century.

Osler, W. (1943) *Aequanimitas.* 3rd ed. New York: Blakiston.

Osler, W. (1951) *Selected Writings: 12 July 1849 to 29 December 1919.* London: Oxford University Press.

Thorn, G.W., Adams, R.D., Braunwald, E. *et al.* eds. (1977) *Harrison's Principles of Internal Medicine.* 8th ed. New York: McGraw-Hill.

Winnicott, D.W. (1949) Hate in the counter-transference. *International Journal of Psychoanalysis,* 30, 69–74.

5

The Ailment[*]

T.F. Main
1957

Editors' reflections

This is one of the most famous papers written about working with difficult service users. It is the paper that most of us read first when trying to understand the dynamics of working with personality disordered individuals, and their effects on staff groups. It remains a widely read and widely cited paper because the clinical description is so good; and most of us can recognise service users we have worked with or colleagues, or even ourselves in the examples given. Tom Main was a group analyst and founded the Cassell Hospital which remains a residential therapeutic community for personality disorder to the present day.

THE AILMENT

When a patient gets better it is a most reassuring event for his doctor or nurse. The nature of this reassurance could be examined at different levels, beginning with that of personal potency and ending, perhaps, with that of the creative as against the primitive sadistic wishes of the therapist; but without any such survey it might be granted that cured patients do great service to their attendants.

---

* Originally published in *British Journal of Medical Psychology*. Thanks to Dr. Main's family for allowing it to be reprinted here.

The best kind of patient for this purpose is one who from great suffering and danger of life or sanity responds quickly to a treatment that interests his doctor and thereafter remains completely well; but those who recover only slowly or incompletely are less satisfying. Only the most mature of therapists are able to encounter frustration of their hopes without some ambivalence towards the patient, and with patients who do not get better, or who even get worse in spite of long devoted care, major strain may arise. The patient's attendants are then pleased neither with him nor themselves and the quality of their concern for him alters accordingly, with consequences that can be severe both for patients and attendants.

We know that doctors and nurses undertake the work of alleviating suffering because of deep personal reasons, and that the practice of medicine, like every human activity, has abiding unconscious determinants. We also know that if human needs are not satisfied they tend to become more passionate, to be reinforced by aggression and then to deteriorate in maturity, with sadism invading the situation, together with its concomitants of anxiety, guilt, depression and compulsive reparative wishes until ultimate despair can ensue. We need not be surprised if hopeless human suffering tends to create in ardent therapists something of the same gamut of feeling.

It is true that he who is concerned only with research and is less interested in therapeutic success than in making findings will not be frustrated by therapeutic failure; indeed, he may be elated at the opportunity for research it provides; but it is not difficult to detect something of the reactions I have described, together with defences of varying usefulness against them. An omnipotent scorn of illness and death, the treatment of patients as instances of disease, the denial of feeling about prognosis, are devices some doctors use to reach at something of the detachment of a research worker, and which permit them to continue their work without too painful personal distress about the frustration of their therapeutic wishes. Refusal to accept therapeutic defeat can, however, lead to therapeutic mania, to subjecting the patient to what is significantly called 'heroic surgical attack', to a frenzy of treatments each carrying more danger for the patient than the last, often involving him in varying degrees of unconsciousness, near-death, pain, anxiety, mutilation or poisoning. Perhaps many of the desperate treatments in medicine can be justified by expediency, but history has an awkward habit of judging some as fashions, more helpful to the amour propre of the therapist than to the patient. The sufferer who frustrates a keen therapist by failing to improve is always in danger of meeting primitive human behaviour disguised as treatment.

I can give one minor instance of this. For a time I studied the use of sedatives in hospital practice; and discussed with the nurses the events which led up to each act of sedation. It ultimately became clear to me and to them that no matter what the rationale was, a nurse would give a sedation only at the moment when she had reached the limit of her human resources and was no longer able to stand the patient's problems without anxiety, impatience, guilt, anger or despair. A sedative would now alter the situation and produce for her a patient who, if not dead, was at least quiet and inclined to lie down and who would cease to worry her for the time being. (It was always the patient and never the nurse who took the sedative).

After studying these matters the nurses recognised that in spite of professional ideals, ordinary human feelings are inevitable, and they allowed themselves freedom to recognise their negative as well as their positive feelings that had hitherto been hidden behind pharmacological traffic. They continued to have permission to give sedatives on their own initiative, but they became more sincere in tolerating their own feelings and in handling patients, and the use of sedatives slowly dropped almost to zero. The patients, better understood and nursed, became calmer and asked for them less frequently.

(This story is, of course, too good to be true, and I have to report that since then occasional waves of increased consumption of aspirin and vitamins have occurred. Such a wave seems to have little to do with patient's needs, for it occurs whenever a new nurse joins the staff or when the nursing staff are overworked or disturbed in their morale.)

The use of treatments in the service of the therapist's unconscious is – it goes without saying – often superbly creative; and the noblest achievements of man in the miracle of modern scientific medicine have all been derived there from. It is deeply satisfying to all mankind that many ailments, once dangerous, mysterious and worrying, now offer the therapist of today wonderful opportunities for the exercise of his skill; but with recalcitrant distress, one might almost say recalcitrant patients, treatments tend, as ever, to, become desperate and to be used increasingly in the service of hatred as well as love; to deaden, placate, and silence, as well as to vivify. In medical psychology the need for the therapist steadily to examine his motives has long been recognised as a necessary, if painful, safeguard against undue obtrusions from unconscious forces in treatment; but personal reviews are liable to imperfections – it has been well said that the trouble with self-analysis lies in the countertransference. The help of another in the review of one's unconscious processes is a much better safeguard, but there can never be certain guarantee that the therapist facing great and resistant distress will be immune from using interpretations in the way nurses use sedatives – to soothe themselves when desperate, and to escape from their own distressing ailment of ambivalence and hatred. The temptation to conceal from ourselves and our patients increasing hatred behind frantic goodness is the greater the more worried we become. Perhaps we need to remind ourselves regularly that the word 'worried' has two meanings, and that if the patient worries us too savagely, friendly objectivity is difficult or impossible to maintain.

Where the arousal of primitive feelings within can be detected by the therapist, he may, of course, put it to good use, and seek to find what it is about the patient that disturbs him in this way. There is nothing new in categorising human behaviour in terms of the impact upon oneself – men have always been able to describe each other with such terms as lovable, exhausting, competitive, seductive, domineering, submissive, etc., which derive from observation of subjective feelings, but the medical psychologist must go further. He must seek how and why and under what circumstances patients arouse specific responses in other human beings, including himself. If only to deepen our understanding of the nature of unconscious appeal and provocation in our patients, we need better subjective observations and more knowledge about the personal behaviour of therapists; and if such observations lead us also to the refinement of medical techniques, so much the better. To use an analogy: it is one sort of observation that some gynaecologists seem to have a need to perform hysterectomies on the merest excuse; it is another that some women seek hysterectomy on the merest excuse. It is not easy to say about a needless hysterectomy which of these is the victim of each other's wishes, which has the more significant ailment, and derives more comfort from the treatment. In a human relationship the study of one person, no matter which one, is likely to throw light on the behaviour of the other.

In the light of those considerations I propose to discuss some events in the hospital treatment of a dozen patients. All were severely ill and before admissions had received treatment at the hands of experts; some had already been in several hospitals and had received many treatments. Further treatment also did little to help them; for none was really well upon discharge from hospital and most were worse. The diagnoses vary from severe hysteria and compulsive obsessional state to depressive and schizoid character disorder. They were admitted at different times over a period of 2½ years, but I came to group them as a class of distinct feature because of what happened. The last of these patients was discharged over five years ago, but I am still ashamed to say that I was pushed into recognising common features by nursing staff who compelled me to take notice of events that had been for long under my nose.

It began this way. The nurses were concerned about a number of their members who had been under obvious strain at their work and sought to know if this could be avoided. It was not a matter of discussing unstable women whose distress could have been regarded merely as personal breakdowns unconnected with work, but rather of valuable colleagues of some sophistication and maturity. The senior nurses met with me to discuss this matter, and I found that they were aware of several episodes of severe individual strain, almost of breakdown, that had occurred over the past three years. I had known of two breakdowns of clinical severity, but I was not aware of these others which had been concealed by the individuals in question. These were now discussed in the open and every case was found to have been associated with the nursing of some particularly difficult patient who had not improved with treatment, and who had been discharged not improved or worse. These patients had been the subject of much discussion during and after their treatment, but even with the passage of time the nurse has been unable to reach a workaday acceptance of the bad prognosis and the failure of treatment. We now found that in spite of having made intensive and praiseworthy efforts with these patients, far in excess of ordinary duty, at least one nurse felt she had failed as a person, and that if only she had tried harder, or known more or been more sensitive, the failure would not have occurred. This feeling ran side by side with another – a resentful desire to blame somebody else, doctor, colleague or relative, for the failure. Each nurse who felt thus was regarded with sympathy and concern by her colleagues as having been associated with patients who were dangerous to the mental peace of their attendants.

It was decided to meet twice a week as a group and to make a retrospective study of all cases which the group listed as major nursing failures. The list contained the dozen names of the patients I mentioned earlier. At that time none of us knew that we were setting out on a trail that was to take us months of painful endeavour to follow.

THE RESEARCH METHOD

At first it was difficult to discuss these patients except by resort to the rather lifeless terms of illness, symptoms and psychopathology, medical and nursing procedures and intentions, and we made little headway. We had yet to discover the potency of group discussion as an instrument of research into relationship with patients. Slowly, following clues in the discussion, the group turned its attention to matters of private feeling as well as professional behaviour with these patients, but this was not easy, especially at first, and many times the group ran into difficulties revealed by silences, depressed inactivity, frightened off-target discussions, and distaste for the investigation by one or more of its members. Sometimes I was able to interpret the difficulty but the other members did so as often. The group was tolerant of the difficulties of its constituent members, and was ready to slow up and wait for anyone who had found the development too fast or the going too heavy, but it stuck to its task and grew the courage step by step to reveal a surprising pattern of old unsettled interpersonal scores hitherto unrecognised by all of us, which had revolved around the nursing of these patients. Private ambitions, omnipotent therapeutic wishes, guilts, angers, envies, resentments, unspoken blamings, alliances and revenges, moves towards and against other nurses, doctors, and patients' relatives, were shown now to have both animated some of the nursing proce-dures offered these patients, and to have been concealed behind them. We had known that these patients had distressed the nurses, and had called forth special effort by them, but we were now astonished to find out how much this was so, and how much feeling and complex social interaction had lain behind the events of patient management.

Each patient had been in hospital for several months and we now turned to study the records of their daily behaviour. From discussion of these the group was able to reconstruct and relive in detail, with more or less pain, the covert configuration of emotions within which these patients had been nursed. We were all aware that the therapeutic passions and intrigues which the group now proceeded to examine with frankness, and more or less pain, were matters of the past, but there was solid agreement – in which I share – that they could not have been examined in vivo and that the truth about them could only be admitted to common awareness after time had allowed feelings to cool and wounds had been licked. We were also agreed that only a group could achieve the capacity to recall past events with the merciless honesty for detail and cor-rections of evasions and distortions that this one required from and tolerated in its members. With each patient discussed, the nurses gave courage to each other and growing insights were used more freely, so that with later cases it was easier for the nurses to recognise and describe the quality of the patients' distress and their own emotional and behavioural responses to it. Finer observations were sometimes made about the later cases, and when this was so, the earlier cases were re-scrutinised for the presence or absence of corresponding phenomena. All findings about any event had to be unanimously agreed by those involved before they were recorded. This led to difficulties when the behaviour of doctors came under discussion, for the group contained none. We now deter-mined to invite the doctor concerned with any case when it was under discus-sion, but this was not a success. The group was now a year old and had grown an unusual capacity for requiring the truth without reserve, and a frankness about emotional involvement with patients, together with a number of sophis-ticated concepts which presented difficulties for anyone who had not shared in the development of the group's work. Moreover, the group was anxious to get on and was no longer as tactful about personal reticence as it had been when it began. One doctor refused the group's invitation, two came once but one declared afterwards that his job was with the patient's psychopathology and not with staff behaviour. (He borrowed the group's findings on one of his patients a year later and lost them.) A fourth came twice and was manfully helpful about his own involvement but was much upset by painful revelations. It must be remembered that these patients were not only nursing, but also medical failures, and as I hope to show, had a remarkable capacity to distress those who looked after then.

The doctors were very, very willing to discuss their patients in terms of psychopathology and of treatment needed and given, but were uneasy when it came to matters of personal feeling. They could not discuss the details of their own difficult personal relationships with these patients, even in obvious instances of which the group was now well aware, except defensively, in terms of self-justification or self-blame. The group was prepared for the doctors to have the same difficulties in discussing old staff mistrusts and covert manoeuvres over patients as they had experienced themselves, and was sympathetic when those proved too great to allow quick collaboration. The nurses already know much about the doctors' behaviour with all of these patients, and, while critical, they were also charitable about it because it had been so similar to their own. It was clear to all how hard the doctors had tried with their patients, had worried, as had the nurses, stifled their disappointments, and made further efforts, and how they, too, had worn themselves to their limit. It was soon clear that it was unfair to expect them to contribute freely about these matters, for they had no opportunity of developing in the group, of sharing in its growth from reticence to frankness, in its pain of overcoming resistances, and its pleasure at finding new ways of viewing their own behaviour. As one nurse said, 'You have to go through it yourself before you can feel easy about what we have found.'

The doctors' views outside the seminar were that these difficult patients needed better diagnosis, better interpretation of ever more primitive feelings, more precise understanding. They, too, were inclined to feel very responsible for the failure of treatment to search for defects in themselves, and to hint at blame of others in the environment – nurses, doctors or relatives.

Now these attitudes were exactly those with which the nurses had begun. The research group had to decide whether to put the brake on its own adventures and wait for the doctors to catch up in sophistication, or to continue without them, with all the deficiencies of information this would mean. The doctors, forewarned of difficulties and of criticism, and lacking the same group need as the nurses to investigate occupational hazards, had also carried more responsibility and were certain to experience prestige problems in the group. These matters would plainly make for heavy going, and, I felt, would complicate an already difficult enough group task. Anyhow, I decided to proceed without their contributions and this account is the poorer thereby. The doctors' troubles with these patients are, however, known in general outline, and at least some features of their behaviour were made plainer.

We proceeded with our survey of hospital events in detail and then came to the question of how far the patients' behaviour had been characteristic not of them but rather of the hospital setting. We therefore surveyed the responses evoked by them in others prior to admission and we made an interesting finding. In hospital, because they had received all sorts of unusual attentions, we had come to refer to them in the group as 'the Special Patients'. Now we found that they had been Special in the eyes of other people before they had come into hospital.

Before I leave the description of the group as a research instrument, using group discussion and scrutiny of records as its method, I must point out one clear gain. The nurses had owned painful distresses, concealed ailments connected with certain patients' ailments, and by disclosing those in respect of themselves and each other, they arrived not only at an increased capacity to recognise insincerities in their daily work, but a personal easement in it. They became less afraid of difficult situations and surer at their craft.

MODE OF ADMISSION

Prior to admission these patients had evoked in their attendants something more than the exercise of practised skills. The referring doctors were level-headed people, some of ripe judgement and deserved reputation, but each felt his patient to be no ordinary person and each asked that she should be given special status and urgent special care. They made special appeals, and in their concern and distress were not content that their patients should be scrutinized and admitted by the ordinary procedures of the hospital. They made almost passionate demands for the waiving of routines because of the patient's distress, and they stressed the special helplessness and vulnerability of the patients in the face of stupid judgements.

The fact that some of these patients had been in mental hospitals and that several had a history of self-destructive acts in the past was mentioned – if at all – not as of warning significance but as an example of former wholly unsuitable handling.

In two cases there was a clear statement that if the patient was not admitted soon, she would have to go to a mental hospital, the implication being that this disastrous step would be all our fault. Great stress was laid on the innate potential of the patient and the pathetic and interesting nature of her illness. Poor prognostic features were concealed or distorted and the group learned to recognise the phrases 'Well worth while' and 'Not really psychotic' as having been ominous special pleas. Personal relationships and past obligations between referrer and hospital doctor were traded upon where present, and four of these cases were first mentioned at friendly social gatherings after the hospital doctor had been offered drinks and a meal by the referrer. In every case the referrer also spoke to the hospital several times by telephone and sent one or more letters.

The referrers had all decided that their patients needed intensive psychotherapy and wished to leave little choice of decision to the hospital. Some seemed to fear that nobody but themselves could really get the hang of the subtleties of feeling in the patient, and that she would be in danger of being judged insensitively as unmanageable rather than 'Special'. Some referrers asked for assurances that she would be handled with extreme care or by a particular doctor.

In all cases, the referrer felt the patient to have been mishandled in the past by other doctors, institutes or relatives, who had been unimaginative or unfeeling, limited in sensitivity, crude rather than culpable; and in there was implied doubt that the hospital staff would have the same limitations.

Many people, doctors, friends, relatives, hospitals and other agencies, had helped in the past, each in their own way, but few were on sincere speaking terms with each other. Most had been impressed with how little real understanding the others had shown and had tried to rescue the patient by giving lengthy unusual services; but all in turn had sooner or later felt that their capacities were beyond their aspirations and had sought somebody better than they, and had begged them to help. As you can imagine, the group called this 'the buck-passing phenomenon', but it was clear that when anyone had handed the patient on, he had done so in apologetic distress, insisting to the patient on his goodwill and that this was for the best, but making it clear that for reasons beyond his control and for which he was not to be blamed, he could do no more. All had felt keenly for the patient, and once the patient was admitted several of the prime helpers wrote letters or visited on her behalf; and letters to them from the patient led them to write to the staff in advisory, pleading or admonitory ways. It was plainly difficult for them to relinquish to others full responsibility for the patient. The research group later made the half-serious conclusion that, whenever the correspondence file of a patient weighed more than 2 lbs, the prognosis was grave.

Our referring doctors were the most recent link of this chain of helpers. They too, had failed to rescue the patient, were uneasy at their failure, and were inclined to blame others, especially relatives, but sometimes colleagues. They were clearly worried by the patient's distress, and wanted to rid themselves of their responsibility, with professions of goodwill. Concern for the patient was emphasised, impatience or hatred never. They asked for help for the patient of the kind they had devised, and wished to leave so little choice to us that it seemed as if we had to be their omnipotent executive organ. It was clear that whatever admission to hospital might do for the patient, it would also do much for them.

In some cases the patient belonged to more than one doctor at once, having gone from one to another without being, or wishing to be, fully relinquished by the first; but there was little consultation between these doctors, and entry into hospital was then less on agreed policy between all doctors and relatives than a determined net by the referrer wishing to rescue the patient from a situation and from people he secretly mistrusted.

All these patients were female. This gives no surprise in a hospital where two-thirds of the patients have always been female, but it may have other significance. Eight were with doctors, doctors' wives, daughters or nieces, or were nurses; a ninth had given blood for transfusion and then because of sepsis had her arm amputated, with great uneasiness among the surgeons concerned. These medical connections are not typical of the unusual hospital admissions, and raise the interesting possibility that there were patients who sought intense relationships with therapists because of their personal past (all of us have heard the story of the doctor's son who said that when he grew up he was going to be a patient). At all events, the referring doctors' freedom of decision was made more complicated by these medical backgrounds, and his prestige in his local medical world was sometimes at stake.

IN HOSPITAL

I shall not describe the patients' personal histories, complaints, symptoms, moods, personal habits, nor the classical diagnostic features of their various states. These were of a kind commonly found in mixed psychiatric practice with severely ill patients, and none explains the nature of the object relations, nor why they, more than other patients with similar diagnosis, became 'Special' and invoked in their attendants so much omnipotence and distress, so great a desire

to help, and so much guilt at the gloomy prognosis. Rather, I will describe
something of their and the staff behaviour.

The last of these patients was discharged five years ago and all concerned
have learned a lot since then, but it would be a mistake to suppose that those
patients were in the hands of beginners, either in psychotherapy or nursing. Of
the seven doctors concerned, at least three would be regarded as experts, two
well trained, and the others as serious apprentices. The nurses were all qualified
but fairly young, and like the doctors, keen to do good work. None of the staff
– this may be a severe criticism – was of a kind that would easily admit defeat.

Each of these patients became 'Special' after they entered the hospital,
some almost at once, others after a month or two. This was not only because of
the referring doctors' wishes, their histories of ill-treatment by others, their
difficult lives or their medical relatives, but because of something in themselves.
Not all severely ill patients are appealing, indeed, some are irritating, but all of
those aroused in the staff, wishes to help of an unusual order, so that the
medical decision to treat the patient in spite of manifestly poor prognosis was
rapidly made. The usual open assessment at staff conference tended to be
quietly evaded, made indecisive or to be regarded as unnecessary; or it was
avoided by the treatment being classified as a special experiment. Each patient
was felt to be a worthwhile person, who had been neglected, who could not be
refused, and who, with special sensitive effort by all, should be given whatever
chance there was without any red-tape nonsense. To every occasion, one or
other of the nursing staff also rose above her best, wishing to make a special
effort to help to rise above 'mere' routines, and to be associated with a compelling case in spite of the extra work it would seem to involve.

It is interesting that under special arrangements each of these patients fairly
quickly acquired special nurses, usually one, occasionally two. Thereafter, this
nurse engaged upon a relationship with the patient that became closer than
usual and both, because of the sharing of crises, became closely in touch with
the therapist outside of the usual treatment sessions or case conferences. These
nurses were regarded by the doctor and the patients and themselves as having a
special feel for the patients' difficulties and a quality of goodness and sensitivity
that was all-important.

The group came to call these features the 'Sentimental Appeal' (from the
patient) and the 'Arousal of Omnipotence' (in the nurse). The nurse thereafter
soon came to feel that she possessed a quality that the others lacked, and began
to protect the patients from unwelcome hospital routines and unwanted visitors
or staff. She would instruct other staff how they should behave towards the
patient and directly or by scheming would ensure that the patient's need for
special privileges or freedom was granted without demur. She would modify or

evade hospital procedures if these were distasteful or upsetting for the patient and be much more permissive and tolerant to special demands than was her usual custom.

The patient's need for special attention was, however, never satisfied except for the shortest periods, so that the nurse was led to demand ever more of herself. She came to feel that distress in the patient was a reproach to insufficiency of her own efforts, so that the handling of her patient became less dictated by her decisions and more by the patient's behaviour. Most of these nurses believed, and were supported by the patient's doctor in their belief, that their efforts for the patient were of great significance, and that by being permissive, even at heavy cost to themselves, they were fulfilling unusual but vital needs in the patient. The nurse usually felt that where others had failed the patient in the past by insensitive criticism, she, by her devotion and attention to the child-like wishes of her patient, could sufficiently still turbulent distress, so that the doctor could better do his work of interpretation. As week after week went by, the patients became more disturbed, but this was seen only as evidence of how ill they always had been basically and how much more devotion they needed than had at first been imagined. The nurse would remain with her patient during panic, anger, depression, or insomnia, soothe her with sedatives, in increasing amounts, protect her from unwelcome situations or unwanted stimuli, ensure that she had special food and accommodation, and special bedtimes, and was given attention immediately she needed it. More time, more sessions, more drugs, more attention, more tact, more devotion, more capacity to stand subtle demand, abuse, ingratitude, insult and spoken or silent reproach was required of the nurse by the patient and by the in-group around her, doctors and colleagues. The patient's wishes, covert rather than overt, were felt to be imperious in that they should stand no delay. Crises occurred of anxiety, depression, aggression, self-destructiveness. The nurse might have on her hands a patient sleepless, importuning and commanding attention, distressed if the nurse wanted to go to the toilet or for a meal, liable to wander cold in her night-dress, perhaps ready to burn herself with cigarettes, bang her head against the wall, cut herself with glass or dash outside. The nurse's time and attention became ever more focussed on the patient so that she would voluntarily spend part of her off-duty, if necessary with the patient. The favourite nurse came to believe, from subtle remarks by the patient that the other nurses, good and effortful though they were, did not have the same deep understanding, so that she would become the patient's unspoken agent, ready to scheme against and control colleagues whose behaviour she felt, through no fault of their own, to be unsuitable for her patient. Increasingly the nurse concerned found herself irresistibly needed by the patient, and sometimes by the therapist, to take over increasing responsibility for some of the patient's ego activities, to think for and decide for the patient, to see that she remembered her appointments with her doctor, fetch and carry, to protect from stimuli, to supervise ordinary bodily functions, such as eating and bathing and lavatory activities. The nurse felt it was woe betide her if she did this badly or forgetfully. To a greater or lesser degree each of those patients ceased to be responsible for some aspect of herself, and with the most severe cases the nurse was expected to diagnose and anticipate the patient's wishes without the patient being put to the trouble of expressing them, to have no other interest than the patient and to be sorry if she failed in this.

There was a queenly quality about some of these patients in the sense that it became for one nurse or other an honour to be allowed to attend them in these exacting ways, and by subtle means the patients were able to imply that unless the nurse did well, favour would be withdrawn, and she would be classed among those others in the world, relatives, previous attendants, etc., who had proved to be untrustworthy and fickle in the past. So skilled were these implications that some nurses became rivals to look after these patients, and felt it as a sign of their own superior sensitivity when the patient finally preferred them to another. The disappointed, unfavoured nurse might feel shame, envy, resentment and sulkily turn elsewhere for other comfort.

The patients were not merely insatiable for attentions such as conversations, interpretations, sedation, hand-holding, time and other things that could be given merely as a matter of duty, they required that these attentions be given with the right attitude and even that the person giving them should do so willingly and with enjoyment. For instance, the nurse would be told, 'You are looking tired', in a tone that was less of concern than of reproach. Or she would be accused after making some considerable effort that she had not enjoyed doing it. Most of these patients were extremely sensitive to negative feelings in their human environment and the group called this 'paranoid sensitivity'. The nurses would at a look of misery from the patient, feel guilty about any reluctance she might have had in providing something for her patient and feel afraid that the patient would detect this. For derelictions of duty or of feeling the nurse might feel punished by the patient becoming turbulent or exposing herself to injury or threatening such a possibility. Nevertheless, there was something about the patients that made nursing them worthwhile.

Behaviour of the same order seems to have occurred with the therapists. Under the stress of treatment they gave unusual services, different from those given to other patients, more devotion, greater effort, with desperate attempts to be good and patient and to interpret the deeper meaning of each of the patient's needs, and to avoid being irritated or suppressive. They, too, felt their extreme worth for the patient. As the patients become more insatiable for attention; more deteriorated in behaviour, restless, sleepless, perhaps aggressive and self-destructive, and intolerant of frustration, the doctor's concern mounted and he was drawn increasingly – except in one case – into advising the nurses on management. The group came to recognise confusion of roles as typical of the situation that grew around and was created by the particular quality of distress in these patients. Therapists accustomed to non-directive roles would give advice on or become active in details of management. Nurses or doctors whose roles were of management only would become minor psycho-therapists during crises, blurring their several roles and professional obliga-tions. Once staff anxiety grew beyond a certain point, therapy became mixed with management, to the detriment of both. The therapist might advise nurses or encourage them to make further efforts, tell them to allow more sedatives if the patient could not sleep, to avoid frustrating the patient in various ways, to carry on sensitively and devotedly and to remain tolerant and friendly. Nurses whom the patient did not like came to be ignored by the therapist and he might try to get the more responsive kind. The nurse thus honoured would be resented by the others who felt hurt by the implications that they were too insensitive.

All those patients had extra treatment sessions over and above the agreed programme, and for some there was grown an arrangement that if the patient were badly distressed in the evening, she or the nurse could telephone the doctor and he would come to the hospital and settle the crisis by giving a session in the patient's bedroom. Increasingly, the therapist accepted his impor-tance for the patient and, showing mistrust of the nurse's ability to manage the patient well, began to take more decisions himself. Having been indulgent with sedatives, some nurses, alarmed at the dosage now required would attempt to get the patient to accept less, but by distressing the doctor, sometimes by telephone, those patients would usually succeed in getting the nurses' decision reversed, until massive doses might be required daily.

The doctor's unusual attentions were, of course, regarded by them as being unorthodox, and they were uneasy that no matter what they did their interpre-tative work did not make the situation better. They pursued their interpretative work ever more intensely and more desperately and continued to do what they could to meet the patient's need for a permissive environment which could tolerate the patient without frustrating her needs. Neurotic diagnoses tended to be altered to psychotic terms and all the illnesses came to be regarded as even more severe than had at first been thought.

Thus, during their stay in hospital, these patients became 'Special', and par-ticular individuals became worn out in the process of attending to their needs.

The patients, appealing at first, and suffering obviously, slowly became insatiable and every effort to help them failed. Nothing given to them was quite enough or good enough, and the staff felt pressed and uneasy that they could not help more. Now this was like the situation that existed prior to admission with the patient and the referring doctor. But, for the Hospital, it was more difficult to pass the case on.

I must now mention some of the effects on the other staff, those not involved, whom I will call the 'Out-group'. These were not principally involved in the treatment of these patients but from time to time cared for them in minor ways on occasions when some member of the 'In-group' was unable to do so. They would be regarded as those whom the patient had not honoured. At first, in open, polite ways, they would disagree that the patient should be handled with special devotion, and sometimes they doubted whether the patient should be handled at all except in a mental hospital. The 'In-group' regarded this view as unworthy (although they did not say so openly), and the 'Out-group' thereafter concealed their opinion and felt unworthy or resentful or even envious of the verve and courage of the 'In-group'. Later, as the patient became worse, the 'Out-group' would become bolder and would discuss among themselves their beliefs that the treatment of this patient was unhealthy, unrealistic, and a waste of time, and later still they would endeavour to keep out of what they felt scornfully, but secretly to be a dangerous and unprofitable situation. They would resent the disturbance the 'Special' patient created for them and their own patients, and then become increasingly critical among themselves of the 'In-group', blaming it for the patient's distress and criticising its handling of the situation as being morbidly indulgent. Stanton and Schwartz (1949a; 1949b; 1949c; 1954) have well described the subsequent fate of the 'In-group'. Under the felt, but undiscussed criticisms it is driven to justify its performance; it withdraws increasingly from contact with the 'Out-group' and concentrates on attending the patient, who, however, only becomes more distressed. Two languages now grow up, one describing the patient as 'getting away with it', 'playing up the staff', 'hysterically demanding'; the other using terms like 'overwhelmed with psychotic anxieties', 'showing the true illness she has hidden all her life', 'seriously ill'. The 'Out-group' now regards the 'In-group' as collusive, unrealistic, over-indulgent, whereas the 'In-group' describes the 'Out-group' as suppressive, insensitive to the strains on an immature ego, lacking in proper feeling. Our research group confirms that this was the case with these patients. The later development of the group situation was agreed to be as follows.

Eventually, the main nurse of the 'In-group' having lost the support of the 'Out-group' and the personal goodwill of colleagues once important to her, and needing, but failing to get justification from her patient's improvement, would become too disturbed to carry on. She would become anxious, or ill, or would suddenly and unexpectedly become angry or in despair with the patient and now feel that it was fruitless to work with such an unrewarding patient or to do good work amid such colleagues. She might say that the patient was far too ill to be nursed outside a mental hospital or might develop the opinion that the patient should be given continuous narcosis or E.C.T., or be considered for a leucotomy. With the growth of unspoken disagreement between the 'In-group' and the 'Out-group' these patients who could sense unspoken tensions unacknowledged by the staff, would get worse and increasingly seek evidence of the reliability and toleration of the 'In-group' and of its capacity to control the 'Out-group'. Then later, when the distress in the 'In-group' mounted, the patient would become panicky, aggressive and self-damaging, demanding and despairing or confused.

The therapist, the centre of the 'In-group', might now, in an effort to preserve his benevolence, advocate the least savage of the physical treatments mentioned, but he might consider others; he might say that he himself was prepared to carry on but felt that the other staff were incapable of giving more, or that because of the risk of suicide the patient should be sent to a closed hospital.

During their stay patients were, in fact, given continuous narcosis and one had a few E.C.T.'s. Four were discharged to closed hospitals, two dying there a year or two after admission from somatic illnesses to which they offered little resistance, one having had a leucotomy. One patient was discharged to an observation ward. One committed suicide in the hospital and another did so after discharge to relatives, who refused advice to send her to a mental hospital. Of five patients discharged home, one later had a leucotomy, three remained in analysis and are leading more stable lives, and the other needed no further treatment.

Even when drawn from 300 patients, such severe failures are dismal. It is true that the previous therapies of these patients – one had been in fifteen hospitals – had failed and that they were all referred as major problems, except one who was thought of as a straightforward neurotic; but failure, after so much effort, is bound to disappoint. These failures did more than disappoint – they left all concerned with mixed feelings of uneasiness, personal blame, and defensive blaming of others. They got under the skin and hurt. Our findings agree with those of Stanton and Schwartz, that certain patients, by having unusual but not generally accepted needs, cause splits in attitudes of the staff, and that these splits, if covert and unresolved, cause the greatest distress to the patients, who could be described as 'torn apart' by them. These two writers warn against easy assumptions that the patient is trying to drive a wedge between staff members, and they point out that the patient's distress can be dramatically resolved if the disagreeing staffs can meet, disclose and discuss their hidden disagreements and reach genuine consensus about how the patient could be handled in any particular matter. We found, however, that the staff splits, while precipitated by disagreements over present events, occurred along lines of feeling and allegiances that had existed prior to the patient coming to hospital. These have too lengthy a history to be described here, but they were complex and hidden from us, until our painful study, under the mask of co-operative feeling by which every community defends itself from disruption. In other words, something about these patients widened and deepened incipient staff splits that would otherwise have been tolerable and more or less unnoticed. Some of the phenomena I have described, particularly the terminal social phenomena, are good examples of the social processes to which Stanton and Schwartz have drawn attention. Their research was not, however, able to include the part played by patients in situations of covert staff disagreement, nor the nature of the patient's wishes. Because of the particular research instrument I came to use – group discussion – I am in a slightly better position to demonstrate the patients' part in increasing incipient disunity. I quote two examples.

One nurse told the research group that there was something about one patient which she alone knew. The patient had told it to her in confidence so that she had felt honoured and trusted more than any other nurse. She had respected the confidence and had spoken to no one about it. It was that the patient had once had a criminal abortion. The group listened to the nurse in silence, and then, first one and then another nurse, revealed that she, too, knew of this, had been told of it in confidence, had felt honoured, and had also felt that the others were too condemnatory to be told about it. We then found that other patients had used similar confidences – which we came to call 'The Precious Little Jewels of Information' – to form special relationships with several nurses, making each feel more knowing than the other, and inhibiting them from communicating honestly with each other. It was as if the patient wanted each one for herself and that each came to want the patient for herself. Thus, split and silenced, each was prepared to be sure that none of the others had the same inner awareness about what was good for the patient, and to feel that the others in their ignorance could only cause distress.

Here, I am reminded of the way in which prior to admission various people had rescued these patients from others whom they mistrusted, and of how often the hospital's sensitivity in turn was mistrusted by the referrer.

My second example concerns a patient whom I visited because of a raised temperature, but whose psychotherapist was another doctor. She was emotionally distressed so I spent longer with her than I had intended and I emerged from my visit with the knowledge that I had a better feel for her emotional difficulties than her own therapist. I realised in all fairness that this was not his fault; for I could not blame him for being less sensitive than I. I then spoke to the patient's nurse and saw from certain hesitations in her account that she believed she had a better feeling for the patient than I had. Each of us believed the other to be lacking in feeling of the special sort needed. I spoke to her of my conjecture and found it to be correct, and we were able thereafter to find out that this patient had made more than ourselves believe that while everybody was doing his or her best, all were really lacking in finer emotions, and only one person in the place was really deeply understanding – oneself.

DISCUSSION

I have had to condense and omit findings such as the large number of minor somatic illnesses that these patients developed, the alarming capacity of at least one to venture, without discoverable physical cause, perilously near the edge of life, and of the way before and after admission people tended to evade telling these patients the full truth if it were painful, but I have given the main outlines of some complex events which merit scrutiny.

I hope it is not difficult to see something of the nature of the distress suffered by the patients' attendants. These patients had an unusual capacity, quite different from that of other patients, to induce not only sympathetic concern but ultimately feelings of massive responsibility arising out of a sense of guilt, one might almost say guilt-by-association with an inconstant untrustworthy and harsh world. This staff guilt grew, and sooner or later, becoming intolerable, was dealt with by denial and by projection on to others: the harsh ones. In addition, denial of guilt was accompanied by compulsive reparative efforts and omnipotent attempts to be ideal. When these efforts failed to still the patient's reproachful distress, further guilt was experienced which, together with hatred, was further denied and projected, and further grand efforts were made at supertherapy. As a persecuting damaged object the patient received frantic benevolence and placating attentions until the controls of increased hatred and guilt in the staff became further threatened. Sedation and other treatments physical and psychological, now came into use almost as coshes to quieten the damaged object that the patient represented. Manoeuvres with and demands for other staff to be kinder and more understanding also began.

Finally, with the cover of staff goodwill cracking, the patient was transferred to other care, or treatment was abandoned, with everyone concerned feeling guilty but continuing to believe in the validity of their own viewpoint and openly or silently blaming the others.

It is to be remembered that these events were hidden and unremarked until difficult study brought then to light, and I believe that similar study of difficult patients in other hospitals' outpatient clinics, private practice and general practice would show similar hidden events. They can be discerned in the behaviour of those who attended these patients prior to admission to hospital, and though these patients are the most gross examples I can find, they are not unique. Whenever something goes wrong with certain distressed patients after lengthy and devoted care, it is not difficult to notice the kind of staff ailment I have described, the sane blaming and contempt of others for their limitations of theory, ability, humanity or realism, and the sane disclaimers of responsibility. Many of you will have no difficulty in recalling problems of managing severely distressed patients, and how often therapists find themselves covertly at odds with professional colleagues with whom they share responsibility, and how the patient goes from one to the other and from one crisis to another. When this happens it is rarely oneself who is wrong-headed, involved or blameworthy, for one is simply doing what one knows to be in the patient's best interests. If, in the words of that convenient phrase, therapy has to be abandoned for external reasons beyond the therapist's control, we cannot help it. We simply did our best in the face of difficulties. With recalcitrant illnesses this end to a therapeutic relationship is far from unknown.

The question to which I now invite your attention is – what is it about such patients that makes for these difficulties? Perhaps there is no general answer, but I offer with hesitation some formulations from existing theory which may be relevant to the features I have described.

The suffering of these patients is noteworthy. Those who had not spent their lives for others as doctors or nurses were worthwhile for other reasons, and the majority could be roughly described as decompensated, creative masochists, who had suffered severely in the past. In her description of a patient whose torturing distress was similar to our patients', Brenman (1952) points out the use made by the masochist of the projection of his own sadistic demands on to objects who are then cared for by self-sacrifice. Others have in somewhat different terms described similar phenomena (Freud, 1937; Klein, 1946). These patients, as their referring doctors said, were or had been or could be worthwhile, that is to say, they had shown some capacity for serving others at cost to themselves. But in none of these women had the defence of projection with masochism succeeded fully, and even before admission their suffering contained marked sadistic elements which were felt and recognised and resented more often by relatives than by doctors. Though they spoke of the world as being impossibly insensitive and demanding, these patients were themselves unremittingly demanding of love, and tortured others to give it by stimulating guilt in them, by self-depreciation and by the extortion of suffering. Self-neglect and helplessness cruelly reproached the world for being no good, and some of them seemed to wish to die in escape from an unproviding world. Tormented by child-like needs and rages, they tormented others also.

The angry response of the 'Out-group' and the readiness for suffering of the 'In-group' may be seen as sadistic and masochistic responses to the sado-masochism of these patients and their raging demands for nurturance, but this is not a complete view.

I am sure you will have noticed their need for material tokens of love and goodwill as well as the eventual insatiability, passion and ruthlessness with which these were pursued. The hostility that reinforced these needs seems to have given rise to features which can be viewed in terms of Melanie Klein's work; fear of the tortured attendant as a retaliating object, appeasement of her by flattery and seduction, demands for more attention as reassurance against the possibility of retaliation. You will note also how these patients isolated and controlled the behaviour of their objects and counter-attacked by savage suffering and appeal when the revengeful potential of their damaged objects seemed great; and how they sought regular reassurance that the object and its goodwill were still alive, reliable and unexhausted. These fruits of aggressive feelings are most easily discernible in the patient's relationship to the nurse, but there is no reason to think that the therapist enjoyed any immunity from them – indeed the evidence is all to the contrary. The more the 'In-group' insisted by its actions that it was not bad or good, the more the patient was beset with the problem of trusting it, and of needing proofs that it was not useless, unreliable and impure in its motives. This in turn further stimulated the staff to deny hatred and to show further good, whereas the patient was beset with the return of her problems in larger size. Thus insatiability grew, and it is interesting to notice that every attention, being ultimately unsatisfying, had to be given in greater amount, poisoned as it was, not only by the patient's motives on the one hand, but by the 'In-group's' hidden ambivalence on the other.

In spite of the fact that the patient frequently feared and attacked the 'In-group', she turned to its strength whenever she felt threatened by other agents. The attempts of the 'In-group' to be all-powerful on her behalf may now be seen as a response to the patient's need to idealise them, and their belief in the badness of the 'Out-group' as their attempt to evade and deflect the patient's projection of sadism. Nevertheless, the 'In-group' itself contained its own problems of mistrust, of finding good and bad among its own members. Mistrust of others made for such confusion in the roles of therapy and management that the nurse could be said to be inhibited not only by her own wishes, but by the wishes of therapists which sometimes contrasted and warred within her. It is only a slight exaggeration to say that at times not only the patient but the nurse was confused about who was who.

Many of the severe panics, depressions, confusions and aggressive outbursts of the patient may thus be viewed as deriving from the sadism that lay behind the suffering in these patients. But, while this explains the later aggressive secondary features, it does not explain naive wishes that were noticeable, especially during the early stages of their therapeutic relations. These wishes were at that stage not aggressive or passionate, but seemed rather to concern an expectation in the patient that was difficult to meet. This simple basic expectation was that someone other than herself should be responsible for her; behind the aggressive use of suffering it was not difficult to see a basic discontent with life and its difficulties. This is found, of course, in all sick and suffering people. In the early stages following admission the nurses were not much tortured by the patient. In addition to all else they were moved by helpless, unspoken and childlike qualities of appeals which became complex only later. The patient's aggressive use of distress can be viewed as sophisticated versions of the signals an infant uses to dominate his mother and bring her to help him. Like infants these patients had a simple, self-centred view of the world – it had to manage them because they could not manage it. Infants need an agent who, in the face of distress, ought to want to diagnose the need and the quality of the satisfaction sought, and the behaviour of our patients with their nurses seemed to contain such needs. The nurse had to undertake responsibility for many of the patients' ego activities which the patients seemed to wish to discard. Some would require her to behave as if she had no identity or biological independence of her own, but was rather a feeling extension of the patient's own body.

The queenly honouring of the nurse with a task that she might regard as difficult is similar to the charming and friendly way a baby will deal with its mother. Anna Freud (1953) has pointed out that, like any parasite, the baby does not excuse his host for her failure but attacks her, reproaches her and demands that she make up for her fault and thereafter be perfect. (I would add here that its queenly love comes first and its displeasure is secondary to imperfections in its host.) The mother is a part of the pair, taken for granted without right to leave, and she has described the baby's sense of the personal loss of part of itself if its mother walks away. If the mother can only give one response (e.g. feeding) for all forms of distress, an addiction to this imperfect response is created for the assuagement of all needs, and this addiction can never be quite satisfying and therefore has to be given forever. The situation can arise out of the mother's limitations, or anxiety, or stupidity, or from her pursuit of theories of child care. Perhaps any theory relentlessly applied creates an addiction.

These patients also fit the description of the early stages of infancy to which Winnicott has given the term pre-ruth. They needed more love than could easily be given and could give little in return except the honour of being cared for. They could be quieted but not satisfied by desperate acts of good will, but they were afraid of the inconstancy of their object, so they would cling to what they had and seek more. The fact that they were aggressive towards and con-temptuous of their objects need not blind us therefore to the fact that needing is an early form of love. But catering for the object's wishes is impossible in the early stages of development prior to what Mrs. Klein calls the depressive position.

Balint (1951) points out that the infant requires his mother not only to be constant and to manage the world and his own body for him in automatic antic-ipation of his wishes, but also to enjoy it and to find her greatest joy in doing so, to experience pain when he is unhappy, to be at one with him in feeling, and to have no other wishes. He goes on to point out that the impossibility of these requirements, except for the shortest periods, leads not only to a disconsolate, forlorn longing for this state, but a fear of the impotent, helpless dependence on the object. Defences therefore arise against the state and its pain in the shape of denial of dependence, by omnipotence and by treating the object as a mere thing. The pain of not being efficiently loved by a needed object is thus defended against by independence; and under the inevitable frustration of omnipotence, hatred of the object for not loving arises. In these patients the need to be at one with the object could be seen in small ways not, to be sure, in the angry, revengeful or domineering behaviour, but in the occasional, early, moving helplessness, in the requests for small satisfaction, in the need for harmony in the relationship and for identity of purpose. The later guilt-driven obedience in their objects was very disturbing to the patients, but I am impressed with the nurses' enjoyment of the earlier simple tasks when both parties could be pleased, the one to give and the other to receive. The nurse truly enjoyed then the honour done her of being accepted by the patient. Smaller enjoyments of this sort also occurred when the patient's simple pleasure might consist of doing some small thing for the nurse. Perhaps it was the rapidly succeeding suspicion of the danger of being helpless and dependent in the future which led the patient to become independent, omnipo-tent and demanding and thus begin the cycle of guilt induction omnipotent care from the nurse, insatiability and suffering.

In drawing attention to these theories of infant behaviour I am in no way suggesting a common psychopathology for the various illnesses from which these patients suffered, and which merit full study in their own right. Rather the possibility arises that certain features of these patients, particularly those which give rise to common behaviour problems, may have primitive origins of a basic order. Nor do I suggest that proper nursing could cure these illnesses, only that the nursing response to these patients and the events of management are crucial moves in a primitive type of object-relation that is strainful for all and which, if not well managed, may become unbearable for all.

The splitting of the staff (including the splitting of the 'In-group') can be thought of as a wedge of the kind a child will drive between its parents but while this explanation will fit the aggressive splitting activities of the patient, it does not fit the fact that, shortly after admission of a patient, the nurses would compete with each other to respond to her silent appealingness. The patient was involved in the split from the first and was later active in maintaining it, but did not seem to cause it in the first place. I am reminded more of the rivalries formed among a group of middle-aged women when a baby whose mother is absent begins to cry, and of the subsequent contest among the women for the honour of being allowed to be of service to it, that is, to be actively distressed by its distress and made actively joyful by its joy. In such an innocent way the baby may evoke rivalries that already existed within such a group in a latent form. It may then become distressed by these rivalries and even make them worse in its search for security, but in the first place it may have wished neither to seek them nor to exploit them. It is true that our patients later become distressed, aggressive and insatiable and then further divided their world in an attempt to control its imperfections, but they were also particularly sensitive to and vulnerable to disharmony in those around them; and, as Stanton and Schwartz have shown, the resolution of felt but undeclared disharmony among their attendants can have a dramatic effect on patients' distress. I would suggest, therefore, that the earliest, but not the later, staff splits were caused by competitive responses in the staff to primitive but impossible appeals from the patient, and that the succeeding hidden competition among the staff led the patient to insecurity and then to the panics, mistrust, demand, hatred and the later active sophisticated splitting activities I have described.

The patient's distress at the splits in the staff may be viewed in terms of the unhappiness experienced by a child whose parents are not on speaking terms and who is made happier by the restoration of a harmonious atmosphere in the home. But it might also be viewed in terms of an infant's distress when in the care of an ambivalent mother, or a mother who misunderstands its needs and pursues, for her own reassurance, authoritative theories on child care. I am inclined to the latter possibility because the splits which distressed these patients contained no sexual preferences and because of their equal distress when receiving ambivalent or determined but inappropriate care by one person, although I realise that this is not a conclusive argument.

The hopelessness, the omnipotent control of the object and the disregard for its purposes may be seen as defence against the dependence of primitive love. Certainly the touchiness, the ruthlessness, as well as the growing insatiability and the mounting sadism that splits the patient's mind and gives rise to confusion, panics, depressions and severe suffering are inherent dangers with these patients. Lastly, I draw attention to the repetitive pattern of the traumatic rejections that beset these patients' lives, both before and after admission and to the possibility that this contains compulsive elements.

SUMMARY AND CONCLUSION

I have described a behaviour syndrome in terms of object relations. Although gross forms are outlined, it is held that minor forms of it can be noted in most medical practice. The patients concerned bore various classic diagnoses, but form a type that cuts across the usual medical classifications and which can be recognised essentially by the object relations formed. This syndrome is difficult to treat successfully, and tends to create problems of management. Further study is needed of its psychopathology, sociology, management and treatment.

The patients suffer severely and have special needs which worry all around them. They tend to exact strained, insincere goodness from their attendants which leads to further difficulties, to insatiability, to a repetitive pattern of eventually not being wanted and to the trauma of betrayal; it also leads to splits in the social environment which are disastrous for the patient and the continuance of treatment.

Sincerity by all about what can and what cannot be given with goodwill offers a basis for management that, however, leaves untouched the basic psychological problems, which need careful understanding, but it is the only way in which these patients can be provided with a reliable modicum of the kind of love they need, and without which their lives are worthless. More cannot be given or forced from others without disaster for all. It is true that these patients can never have enough, but this is a problem for treatment and not for management.

It is important for such patients that those who are involved in their treatment and management be sincere with each other, in disagreement as well as agreement, that each confines himself to his own role, and that each respect and tolerate the other's limitations without resort to omnipotence or blame. It is especially important for each to avoid the temptation to induce others into becoming the executive instruments of his own feelings and wishes.

It is customary in a Chairman's address to seize the rare occasion when tradition rules that there be no disaster, to proffer advice. Believing that sincerity in management is a sine qua non for the treatment of the patients I have described, I offer the Section one piece of advice. If at any time you are impelled to instruct others to be less hostile and more loving than they can truly be – don't!

I cannot conclude without paying tribute to the nurses and doctors who allowed me to share the study of their difficult work and to the pleasure I have had with them in formulating these ideas.

REFERENCES

Balint, M. (1951) On Love and Hate, Primary Love and Psycho-Analytic Technique. London: Hogarth Press and Institute of Psycho-Analysis.

Brenman, M. (1952) On Teasing and Being Teased, and the Problem of 'Moral Masochism'. Psychoanalytic Study of Children, 7.

Freud, A. (1937) The Ego and the Mechanisms of Defence. London: Hogarth Press and Institute of Psycho-Analysis.

Freud, A. (1953) Some Remarks on Infant Observation. Psychoanalytic Study of Children, 8.

Klein, M. (1946) 'Notes on some Schizoid Mechanisms.' In M. Klein, P. Heimann, S. Isaacs and J. Riviere (eds.) Developments in Psycho-Analysis. London: Hogarth Press, 1952.

Stanton, A.H. and Schwarz, M.S. (1949a) The Management of a Type of Institutional Participation in Mental Illness. Psychiatry, 12, 13, 26.

Stanton, A.H. and Schwarz, M.S. (1949b) Medical Opinion and the Social Context in the Mental Hospital. Psychiatry, 12, 243–9.

Stanton, A.H. and Schwarz, M.S. (1949c) Observations on Dissociation as Social Participation. Psychiatry, 12, 339–54.

Stanton, A.H. and Schwarz, M.S. (1954) The Mental Hospital. New York: Basic Books.

6

Malignant Alienation: Dangers for Patients Who are Hard to Like*

Darryl Watts and Gethin Morgan
1994

· ·

Editors' reflections

The next classic paper reminds us that working with personality disorder means working with people who have mood disorders. There is massive overlap between personality disorder and depression, especially in cases of borderline personality disorder, and the risk of suicide is ever present, even if it waxes and wanes in intensity. What is particularly good about this paper is that it is a reminder that personality disorder is about interpersonal dysfunction: that the suicidal service user feels alienated from other people, often especially those who are in a caring role. This paper also reminds us that suicidal people often induce hatred and rejection, rather than sympathy: they can induce in us that same loathing that they have for themselves. See also Mary Whittle's paper about malignant alienation in a forensic setting.

· ·

MALIGNANT ALIENATION

The assessment and management of suicide risk are among the most difficult clinical skills to acquire. Seager and Flood (1965) examined coroners' inquisi-

---

* Originally published in *British Journal of Psychiatry*, *164*, 11–15. Reprinted here by permission of The Royal College of Psychiatrists.

tions on 325 suicides which occurred during 1957–61 and found that 4.6% had taken place during in-patient or day-psychiatric care, and 16% within six months of receiving such treatment. More recent work confirms the relatively common occurrence of suicide in spite of close psychiatric supervision. In Avon, 29% of all those committing suicide had been seen by a psychiatrist at some time during the previous year (Vassilas, 1993; personal communication). Clearly, much remains to be done in improving techniques of predicting suicide risk and in its management.

Sociodemographic, medical and psychiatric risk factors which may predict suicide have been well documented (Hawton, 1987). These are most useful with regard to long-term risk, but what the clinician needs primarily is guidance on how to identify those at immediate high risk. Relatively little attention has been paid to the systematic evaluation of day-to-day behaviour and relationship with others in the detection of such short-term risk.

Alienation in particular seems worthy of careful attention. Truant *et al.* (1991) surveyed psychiatrists in London, Ontario, and found that 61% of respondents believed that those patients who were rejected, isolated or detached were more likely to commit suicide. Three of the top eight selected risk factors were in the category 'quality and continuity of interpersonal relationships'.

Morgan (1979) coined the term 'malignant alienation' to describe a process which appeared to have been common before suicide in a small series of psychiatric in-patients. It was characterised by a progressive deterioration in their relationship with others, including loss of sympathy and support from members of staff, who tended to construe these patients' behaviour as provocative, unreasonable, or overdependent. In some instances an element of deliberately assumed disability was invoked. Such alienation between patient and others appeared to have been malignant in that it gained momentum and was associated with a fatal outcome (Morgan and Priest, 1984). A further study of suicides among psychiatric patients in Bristol (Morgan and Priest, 1991) showed that the process of alienation was a theme in 55% of such deaths.

COMPONENTS OF MALIGNANT ALIENATION

It is convenient to discuss the important components in malignant alienation in four parts: patient factors, staff factors, staff–patient interaction, and hospital environment.

Patient factors

As part of a research project with the National Institute of Mental Health, Fawcett *et al.* (1969) studied 30 depressed suicidal patients at varying risk of suicide. Patients' interpersonal behaviour on the ward was documented, along with interpersonal behaviour before the illness (obtained from interviews with spouses/family and records of joint interviews). They identified four factors indicative of the quality of long-standing interpersonal relationships that discriminated a high-risk group from the remainder. These were: interpersonal incapacity (a lifelong inability to maintain warm, mutually interdependent relationship); marital isolation (interpersonal isolation and disengagement in spite of overt appearances of a conventional marriage, i.e. emotional divorce); distorted communication of dependency wishes (an inability to express directly dependency needs which might lead to support); and help negation (persistent withdrawal or denial of helpful relationships). The authors felt this supported the hypothesis that the depressed patient at high risk of suicide had a long-standing inability to communicate wishes/needs effectively, predating the index illness. It is unlikely that these results are specific to a depressed suicidal group.

Henderson (1974) looked at the concept of care-eliciting behaviour from phylogenetic and ontogenetic perspectives. Normal care-eliciting serves important functions: survival of the infant initially (cf. attachment theory) and the maintenance of strong social bonds in adulthood. Pathological care-eliciting stands separately only insofar as it is disruptive for the individual, or would-be carer, or both. The signals used (e.g. parasuicide, conversion hysteria, factitious disorders, shoplifting) may cause distress to self or carer, but their consequence is developmentally ancient: they bring others closer.

However, there is the risk of exceeding the limits of tolerance of the carers. In addition, abnormal care-eliciting tends to evoke ambivalent responses in carers. According to Parsons (1951), adoption of the sick role is permissible only when the disability is considered genuine and the patient cooperates in efforts towards a return to health. Otherwise there is an infringement in the code relating to illness behaviour, a code held particularly strongly by health-care professionals. The converse of our particular social code relating to illness was clearly pointed out by Samuel Butler (1872) in his novel Erewhon – where to be ill was to be punished but to be dishonest attracted care and sympathy.

Staff factors

Hospital staff may bring with them unrealistic expectations and aspirations for care giving. These vulnerabilities have been termed 'narcissistic snares' (Maltsberger and Buie, 1974), and may be universal among less experienced or poorly supervised staff. The three commonest snares are the aspirations to 'heal all, know all and love all'. These can be compounded by the magical hopes of the patient at the beginning of treatment, when carers may become infected with expectations of omnipotence. Clearly, the risk for carers is in finally feeling helpless, guilty and wishing themselves far from the patient.

Psychiatric health-care professionals are particularly prone to expectations of healing all, for two reasons. Firstly, the personality of the carer is often the therapeutic tool, unlike surgery or medicine where the means of treatment are simpler to separate from the self. Thus the psychiatric carer confuses professional capacity to heal with a sense of self-worth. Secondly, change in psychiatric patients often occurs slowly, frustrating the drive of those ardent to see improvement.

The expectation for omniscience is as much a snare. The experienced psychiatrist does not follow intuition beyond a certain point and hunches are constantly examined against the clinical evidence. Following one's empathic sense alone as to whether a patient is suicidal or not can be fatal.

The third snare is that the carer should love all. Unfortunately, objectivity can be compromised in an attempt to be seen as a caring person – particularly with patients whose transference will involve denouncement of the carer as cold or uncaring. The carer is left open to attack on a disposition to lovingness. Once breached, this brittle defence may crumble, leaving the carer feeling initially helpless, then retaliatory.

Staff–patient interaction

In many staff, strong negative feelings may be provoked by patients. Knowing which patients provoke these feelings and how staff deal with the feelings is crucial to understanding the alienation process.

Colson *et al.* (1985) examined which patients are perceived by staff as 'difficult to treat'. This concept is important, as the staff's view of a patient as difficult to treat may exert a powerful influence on the patient, the carers and the treatment process, with implications for progress and prognosis. Four symptom clusters were found that related to staff perception of treatment difficulty, and also to perceived poorer progress and prognosis. In descending order of influence the factors were: withdrawn psychoticism, severe character pathology, suicidal depressed behaviour, and violence/agitation.

It is suggested that patients with these characteristics interact in a particular way with staff. Perhaps psychotically withdrawn patients (regressed, withdrawn, isolated, bizarre) are experienced as most difficult to treat because they are difficult to engage and inaccessible to interpersonal intervention. The patient with severe character pathology (demanding, plays one person against another, manipulative, moody) may repel staff by the intense and troublesome contact made. The behaviour of the suicidal depressed patient (self-abusive, depressed, regression after progress) is seen as difficult to treat because of the patient's tendency to react to the prospect of progress with depressive feelings of defeat.

This points to the crucial containing role of the therapeutic alliance with difficult patients, and how problems could arise if the alliance fails, or cannot be formed. The therapeutic alliance may have a protective role, protecting patients from the strong negative feelings engendered in staff when patients are perceived as difficult to treat.

Perhaps the most difficult provoked feeling to contain is hate. Some patients are unable to contain their own hate for a needed person (e.g. parent, nurse or doctor). Instead, the hate is projected and the patient feels better as responsibility for the hatred is shared ('I hate him and he hates me') and anxiety reduced ('You hate me so my hate for you is justified'). Direct and indirect means are then used to provoke carers' hate, to substantiate the projection. Abusive, disparaging language, sullen silence, repeated somatic complaints or forgotten appointments may all kindle the ire of carers (Maltsberger and Buie, 1974).

Countertransference is inevitable in all patient contact. In its broadest sense it means the carer's emotional response to the patient, stemming from both the specific carer–patient relationship and the disposition of the carer. Conscious countertransference can usually be controlled, and may shed light onto details of the patient previously hidden. Unconscious countertransference may give rise to well rationalised but destructive acting out by carers.

Countertransference hate may be found at the heart of the malignant alienation process, and deserves attention. Countertransference hate has two components: malice and aversion (Maltsberger and Buie, 1974). While carers find the malicious component harder to tolerate, it is the aversion which is most dangerous to the patient. The carer's malicious feelings imply a preservation of the relationship with the patient, whereas the aversive impulse tempts the carer to abandon the patient. It is this abandonment (alienation on the ward, premature discharge, transfer), which has lethal potential. Paradoxically, the temptation is to abandon the patient in order not to bear the countertransference malice.

The internal economy of countertransference hate in carers consists of a subtle balance between defensive postures and conscious awareness. Of course, carers are compassionate and non-judgemental, and do not vent punitive, rejecting, murderous or disgusted feelings on patients. However, carers are human, and have the potential for these feelings, although it is individually difficult to admit to them. Intolerance of the hateful countertransference may also explain its absence from standard psychiatric textbooks.

The defences used to prevent conscious awareness of countertransference hate include repression, reaction formation, projection, and distortion/denial. Repressing the feelings is relatively safe for the patient, but the carer may convey aversion/hostility by non-verbal messages such as clockwatching, inattentiveness or yawning.

The other defences can have lethal consequences for the patient. With reaction formation (turning the countertransference hate into the opposite), the carer is oversolicitous, experiences an anxious drive to help, and meddles. Like an overindulgent parent, the carer may overprescribe and overhospitalise. Projecting the countertransference hate ('I do not wish to kill you, you wish to kill yourself') is experienced by the carer as a dread that the patient will commit suicide, no matter what. This can lead either to imposition of unnecessary controls (as if to 'provoke' the suicide), or to rejection of a 'hopeless case' (if the aversive element dominates). The mute, suicidal patient is particularly likely to become the target of projected countertransference hate. To sit for hours with such rejecting patients can evoke hateful fantasies. Distortion/denial is another route to impaired judgement on the part of the carer, who selectively attends to the facts of the clinical situation in order to repudiate and devalue the patient. The patient is seen as a hopeless case, or a dangerous person. There is a lack of basic respect for the patient as the carer experiences indifference and finally rejects the patient.

Hospital environment

In a benchmark paper, Winnicott (1949) likened caring for the psychotic or difficult patient to a mother caring for a demanding baby:

> However much he loves his patients he cannot avoid hating them and fearing them, and the better he knows this the less will hate and fear be the motives determining what he does to his patients.

Winnicott saw this hate as normal, but pointed out that particular aspects of the hospital environment are not conducive to openness about hate; such openness may be seen as professionally unacceptable, and unsafe (for both staff and patients) to express openly, and patients may be regarded as too ill for staff to let them know how much they are hated. However, without some recognition in hospital, the hateful feelings will be sublimated or projected elsewhere. In addition, the staff may not be 'good enough parents', able to be hurt while hating so much, without payback (acting out of countertransference hate), and able to wait for rewards. If rewards do not come (the patient does not improve and go home), then there is the risk of payback. As Winnicott suggests, 'Down will come baby, cradle and all.' Essentially, there may not be the culture in psychiatric hospital wards necessary to discuss openly these powerful negative feelings.

MALIGNANT ALIENATION – A SYNTHESIS

We suggest the above factors all play a part in a particular process, the terminal phase of which is called malignant alienation. Real benefits in the clinical care of psychiatric patients could accrue from understanding the process in the following way.

Patients involved in this process may have longstanding problems in communicating their needs effectively, attempting instead to have their care needs met in less appropriate ways. These patients may have infringed the 'sick-role' code, claiming illness without cooperating in attempts to return to health, perhaps in the absence of understandable disability. This provokes an ambivalent response in carers. The patients perceived as difficult to treat can be described as withdrawn, psychotic, having severe character pathology, suicidally depressed, or the violent/agitated. In common there is a poor, unformed or failed treatment alliance, which is unable to contain these perceived treatment difficulties.

In addition, carers are often unaware of their own vulnerabilities (narcissistic snares), and may work in a culture not generally receptive to open discussion of the powerful negative feelings generated. At the end, with only a shaky therapeutic alliance, countertransference hate remains unconscious, and is acted out by carers towards the patient. The difficult patient is alienated and finally placed at high risk of suicide.

STRATEGIES FOR PREVENTING AND MANAGING MALIGNANT ALIENATION

Certain clinical strategies may be useful in preventing and managing the alienation process. These may be itemised as follows:

(a)   Equating challenging behaviour with an inability to seek help in other ways, and acknowledgement of the patient's possible inner distress.

(b)   Promoting a ward environment in which any negative feelings among staff members can be acknowledged openly at staff meetings and ideally at support groups (this aspect of clinical work should be an essential ingredient of effective supervision: staff members should be helped to acknowledge, bear, and put into perspective their countertransference hate).

(c)   Providing insight into staff members' own vulnerabilities and expectations in providing care provision (such self-awareness is vital in those who have a need to develop special close relationships with certain patients and who encourage close dependency).

(d)   Early identification of those patients whom staff perceive as failing to improve, particularly when there are demands from staff for their discharge from care (setting limits of patient behaviour is an important strategy in clinical care but requires scrupulous assessment of the reasons why they should be implemented).

(e)   Early identification of a lack of therapeutic alliance.

(f)   Providing post-recovery conjoint sessions with a spouse or other significant person for those patients who have particular difficulty in communicating their needs effectively (exclusion of significant others in the management of suicide risk may itself be hazardous).

It may also be possible to extend these ideas out of the psychiatric hospital ward and into other caring environments where malignant alienation could occur. The prevention and management of the malignant alienation process in potentially suicidal patients may have close analogy with the psycho-social intervention which has been shown to be effective at preventing relapse in schizophrenic patients whose close relatives exhibit high expressed emotion (Leff *et al.* 1985).

THE PRESENT SCENE

A thorough understanding of malignant alienation is particularly important at the present time as new styles of psychiatric services place increasing emphasis on care in the community (Morgan, 1992). While such developments are commendable, the process of change must depend upon an appropriate balance between in-patient and community facilities. Regrettably, in-patient units are often greatly reduced in size before community resources have been developed adequately. The resulting need for rapid discharge will make it even more difficult to assess adequately the needs of patients at risk of suicide. The process of malignant alienation then becomes an even greater hazard unless facilities in the community really can assume functions lost from in-patient provision. Establishment of community care should not be at the expense of providing help for the difficult, the awkward, and the demanding, who at times may need protection from the negative, aggressive aspects of ourselves (Hill, 1978).

ACKNOWLEDGEMENT

The authors wish to thank Dr John Lambourn for useful discussions.

REFERENCES

Butler, S. (1872) *Erewhon*. London: Trubner and Co.

Colson, D.B., Allen, J.G., Coyne, L., *et al.* (1985) Patterns of staff perception of difficult patients in a long-term psychiatric hospital. *Hospital and Community Psychiatry*, 36, 168–172.

Fawcett, J., Leff, M. and Bunney, W.E. (1969) Suicide: Clues from interpersonal communication. *Archives of General Psychiatry*, 21, 129–137.

Hawton, K. (1987) Assessment of suicide risk. *British Journal of Psychiatry*, 150, 145–153.

Henderson, S. (1974) Care-eliciting behaviour in man. *Journal of Nervous and Mental Disease*, 159, 172–181.

Hill, D. (1978) The qualities of a good psychiatrist. *British Journal of Psychiatry*, 133, 97–105.

Leff, J., Kuipers, L., Berkowitz, R., *et al.* (1985) A controlled trial of social intervention in the families of schizophrenic patients: Two year follow-up. *British Journal of Psychiatry*, 146, 594–600.

Maltsberger, J.T. and Buie, D.H. (1974) Countertransference hate in the treatment of suicidal patients. *Archives of General Psychiatry*, 30, 625–633.

Morgan, H.G. (1979) *Death Wishes: The Understanding and Management of Deliberate Self Harm*. Chichester: Wiley.

Morgan, H.G. (1992) Suicide prevention: Hazards on the fast road to community care. *British Journal of Psychiatry*, 160, 149–153.

Morgan, H.G. and Priest, P. (1984) Assessment of suicide risk in psychiatric in-patients. *British Journal of Psychiatry*, 145, 467–469.

Morgan; H.G. and Priest; P. (1991) Suicide and other unexpected deaths among psychiatric in-patients. The Bristol confidential inquiry. *British Journal of Psychiatry*, 158, 368–374.

Parsons, T. (1951) *The Social System*. Glencoe: The Free Press.

Seager, C.P. and Flood, R.A. (1965) Suicide in Bristol. *British Journal of Psychiatry*, 111, 919–932.

Truant, G.S., O'Reilly, M.B. and Donaldson, L. (1991) How psychiatrists weigh risk factors when assessing suicide risk. *Suicide and Life-Threatening Behaviour*, 21, 106–114.

Winnicott, D.W. (1949) Hate in the Countertransference. *International Journal of Psychoanalysis*, 30, 69–74.

7

Malignant Alienation[*]

Mary Whittle
1997

. . . .

Editors' reflections

This paper takes Watts and Morgan's original paper and applies it specifically to the forensic service-user population. Whittle highlights the therapeutic challenges faced by both staff and service users in forensic settings in relation to stigma, especially when the word 'difficult' becomes associated with the service user's identity. Malignant alienation in the forensic context describes the process whereby forensic service users evoke especially malignant countertransferential feelings in staff. All forensic staff struggle with these feelings (which include shame, disgust, excitement and fear), and this struggle can lead to breakdown of the therapeutic alliance. However, malignant alienation in a forensic context also refers to the process whereby individuals project their own malignant feelings towards themselves into staff, or the institution. Such projections can lead to staff or the institution withdrawing and neglecting the service user's distress. This may explain the high levels of suicidal behaviour or completed suicide in forensic settings. Therefore, it is those service users who are the most resistant to treatment, and most attacking of help, that require the most reflection and attention to avoid the trap of malignant alienation.

. . . .

[*] Originally published in *Journal of Forensic Psychiatry and Psychology*, 8, 1, 5–10. Reprinted here by permission of Taylor and Francis.

'Malignant alienation' describes a process of deterioration in relationships with staff which precedes suicide in a number of patients (Morgan, 1979; Morgan and Priest, 1984). Interaction of factors in the patient, staff and hospital environment is linked with failure of the therapeutic alliance (Watts and Morgan, 1994); staff perceive the patient as difficult, provocative and manipulative. Criticism and hostility towards the patient increase in the period before the suicide. Alienation of the patient is considered malignant as the process is progressive and associated with the death of the patient.

The possibility exists that patients also experience alienation that has seriously detrimental associations (i.e. is malignant) but is not linked with suicide. In a study of four psychiatric hospitals, one-fifth of patients felt that staff considered them a nuisance (Myers et al., 1990). Evidence for critical and hostile attitudes (and actions) towards patients has often emerged from forensic institutions. Harmful consequences for patients have not only been associated with suicide but also included physical and sexual abuse and death following enforced medication (Lipsedge, 1994; Secretary of State for Health, 1992).

Forensic patients may be particularly vulnerable to malignant alienation. Self-harm is common among forensic patients (Maden et al., 1993; Powell et al., 1994). Referral to forensic services may occur as part of an alienation process (Mullen, 1993). The nature of the patients' offences or fears for personal safety may provoke disgust and aversion. The sobriquet of 'difficult' preceding a patient may prime negative attitudes in staff.

Patients who are 'difficult' to manage are found commonly among the patients of maximum secure hospitals (Maden et al., 1993) and account for one-third of referrals to regional forensic services (Mendelson, 1992). Staff perceive difficult patients as dangerous and have difficulty empathizing with them. They provoke fear, anger, helplessness and polarization in staff. They are likely to be severely ill, to have more diagnoses and to receive unnecessary medication (often despite awareness of their poor compliance with or abuse of medication) (Neill, 1979). Antisocial and aggressive features, self-mutilation, sexual deviations and drug addiction are common (Ekdawi, 1967). Labels associated with 'difficult' patients, i.e. 'obnoxious' (Groves, 1978), 'hostile', 'unpredictable', 'demanding', 'complaining' and 'argumentative' (Ekdawi, 1967; Flood and Seager, 1968), are similar to those of malignant alienation.

Failure of the therapeutic alliance is a key factor in the development of malignant alienation (Watts and Morgan, 1994). Good therapeutic alliance is associated with utilization of treatment resources, compliance with drug treatment (Kaminstein, 1989; Frank and Gunderson, 1990) and improved therapeutic outcome (Allen et al., 1985; Clarkin et al., 1987; Frank and Gunderson, 1990). The developing and maintaining of a therapeutic alliance imply that the patient accepts the need for treatment and is able to trust, and be willing to work with, the therapist towards the resolution of his or her problems (Sandier *et al.*, 1970). Some forensic patients are reluctant participants, forced into therapeutic relationships by detention or treatment orders. Hostility, though not precluding the development of a positive therapeutic alliance (Sandier *et al.*, 1970), must be overcome. Many forensic patients with chronic psychiatric disability lack insight into their problems (Maden *et al.*, 1993). The improved therapeutic alliance associated with clinical improvement (Allen *et al.*, 1985) will be of little benefit to patients with refractory conditions. Patients with psychosis and those who experienced severe emotional deprivation in childhood may have difficulty in forming the trusting relationship needed for a successful treatment alliance (Sandier *et al.*, 1970). 'Likeability', i.e. aspects of the patient such as personal charm and ability to evoke the interest of staff, is correlated with treatment alliance (Allen *et al.*, 1985) and may be compromised by the nature of the patients' offences. Patients often find it difficult to develop treatment alliances with a large group of carers at once (Allen *et al.*, 1985) and those who have problems in communicating effectively with others or who seek help only in maladaptive ways risk exceeding the tolerance of staff (Henderson, 1974; Valliant, 1992). Substance abuse has been linked with poor treatment alliance in hospitalized patients (Clarkin *et al.*, 1987) and is common among forensic patients.

Therapist factors also affect the therapeutic alliance. The forensic psychiatrist should demonstrate 'tolerance for difficult patients', free himself or herself of 'moralistic judgements…and not allow emotional attitudes to interfere with clinical judgements' (Chiswick and Cope, 1995). Such statements set standards against which to assess ourselves and our practice but minimize the complexity of relationships between staff and patients in forensic institutions. It is ingenuous to suggest that staff–patient relationships occur in situations of complete tolerance, free from emotional attitudes and moral judgement. This is not to say that staff are not constantly striving towards these ideals but to argue that complex interactions occur at conscious and unconscious levels in both patients and staff. Factors in staff which promote or hinder the development or maintenance of the therapeutic alliance should, therefore, be kept under review.

Transference and countertransference are unavoidable in patient–therapist relationships (Adler, 1972; Maltsberger and Buie, 1974; Hill, 1978) and affect the therapeutic alliance. Unrecognized negative countertransference is associated with suicide (Modestin, 1987), splitting of the treatment team, breakdown in professional communication and the delivery of inadequate care (Maltsberger, 1995). Misdiagnosis, mistreatment and the compromise of professional skills ensue from denial or suppression of negative or hateful feelings about patients (Groves, 1978). Countertransference hate plays an important part in malignant alienation (Watts and Morgan, 1994). The therapist who experiences countertransference hate cannot avoid hating and fearing the patient despite caring for him or her (Winnicott, 1949). Action by the therapist based on the malice and aversion components of countertransference hate can lead to rejection, premature discharge or transfer of the patient (Maltsberger and Buie, 1974).

It is possible that a mismatch between the personal feelings of staff, the professional etiquette that prohibits the expression of negative feelings towards patients, and the limited range of institutional responses to provocative behaviour (such as medication or seclusion for self-harming or violent behaviour (Norton and Dolan, 1995), may provoke staff to reduce contact with certain patients. Escalation of violent behaviour may ensue as severely disturbed patients attempt to gain attention when levels of staff–patient inter-action are low (Drinkwater, 1982). The need to care for the patient may encourage unrealistic expectations by staff that they can tolerate and treat all aspects of the patient. Such hopes are likely to be dashed, disappointing the carer and facilitating negative countertransference towards the patient (Maltsberger and Buie, 1974; Watts and Morgan, 1994).

Staff in forensic units work in situations where violence is common (Torpy and Hall, 1993) and attacks on persons or property must be dealt with effec-tively to ensure safety (Maltsberger and Buie, 1974; Valliant, 1992). While not underestimating the difficulties faced by staff in managing violent behaviour, we need to acknowledge that the threat of personal violence may precipitate stress and cloud judgement (Whittington and Mason, 1995). In these situa-tions, acting on negative countertransference by staff can take a variety of forms, e.g. unwarranted or prolonged use of seclusion, inappropriate changes in diagnosis, delay in admitting difficult patients, or precipitous decisions to return patients to prison. Hospital cultures in which staff are professionally isolated, and which lack openness, scrutiny or staff support systems, risk the creation of a medium in which malignant alienation can flourish (Secretary of State for Health, 1992; Mullen, 1993; Watts and Morgan, 1994).

The grave consequences of malignant alienation behove us to prevent it. Developing a treatment alliance needs time (Frank and Gunderson, 1990) and staff require support to build relationships with patients whose behaviour is disturbed, threatening or antisocial. Problems in the therapeutic alliance must be identified and dealt with as early as possible. Particular attention should be paid to patients who are perceived as failing to improve or for whom limit setting or discharge is at issue (Watts and Morgan, 1994). The risk of alienation will decrease if staff equate challenging behaviour with maladaptive attempts to seek help (Watts and Morgan, 1994) and assist patients in finding more adaptive ways of communicating their distress. Exploration of patients' strengths and personal interests could reduce negative stereotyping, which has been associated with the death of patients following enforced medication (Lipsedge, 1994).

Staff who have little training can exert considerable influence on prevailing attitudes (Scott and Philip, 1985) and it is possible for hostile or critical attitudes to develop in staff of all disciplines and experience who have contact with patients. With suitable training and supervision, simple psychotherapeutic techniques can be used fruitfully by any mental health worker to improve relationships with patients (Wieden and Havens, 1994). It must be made easy for staff to express feelings about patients and gain insights into their own vulnerabilities and expectations as carers in a well supervised, supportive environment (Watts and Morgan, 1994).

Forensic psychiatric patients are among the most challenging patients cared for by mental health workers. Awareness of malignant alienation would assist staff to improve quality of care and reduce the risk of abusive behaviour with this demanding and vulnerable group of patients.

REFERENCES

Adler, G. (1972) Helplessness in the Helpers. *British Journal of Medical Psychology*, 45, 315–25.

Allen, J.G., Tarnoff, G. and Coyne, L. (1985) Therapeutic Alliance and Long-term Hospital Treatment Outcome. *Comprehensive Psychiatry*, 26(2), 187–94.

Chiswick, D. and Cope, R. (1995) *Practical Forensic Psychiatry*. London: Gaskell.

Clarkin, J.R., Hurt, S.W. and Crilly, J.L. (1987) Therapeutic Alliance and Hospital Treatment Outcome. *Hospital and Community Psychiatry*, 38(8), 871–5.

Drinkwater, J. (1982) 'Violence in Psychiatric Hospitals'. In P. Feldman. (ed.) *Developments in the Study of Criminal Behaviour*. Vol. II, *Violence*. Chichester, Sx: Wiley. Pp.111–130.

Ekdawi, M.Y. (1967) The Difficult Patient. *British Journal of Psychiatry*, 113, 547–52.

Flood, R.A. and Seager, C.P. (1968) A Retrospective Examination of Psychiatric Case Records of Patients Who Subsequently Committed Suicide. *British Journal of Psychiatry*, 114, 451–7.

Frank, A.E. and Gunderson, J.G. (1990) The Role of the Therapeutic Alliance in the Treatment of Schizophrenia. *Archives of General Psychiatry*, 47, 228–36.

Groves, J.E. (1978) Taking Care of the Hateful Patient. *New England Journal of Medicine*, 298(16), 883–7.

Henderson, S. (1974) Care-Eliciting Behaviour in Man. *Journal of Nervous and Mental Disease*, 159, 172–81.

Hill, D. (1978) The Qualities of a Good Psychiatrist. *British Journal of Psychiatry*, 53, 97–105.

Kaminstein, P. (1989) Importance of the Transference and Therapeutic Alliance in Pharmacotherapy (letter). *American Journal of Psychiatry*, 146(3), 404–5.

Lipsedge, M. (1994) Dangerous Stereotypes. *Journal of Forensic Psychiatry*, 5(1), 14–19.

Maden, A., Curie, C., Meux, C., Burrow, S. and Gunn, J. (1993) The Treatment and Security Needs of Patients in Special Hospitals. *Criminal Behaviour and Mental Health*, 3, 290–306.

Maltsberger, J.T. and Buie, D.H. (1974) Countertransference Hate in the Treatment of Suicidal Patients. *Archives of General Psychiatry*, 30, 625–33.

Maltsberger, J.T. (ed.) (1995) Case Consultation. Diffusion of Responsibility in the Care of a Difficult Patient. *Suicide and Life-Threatening Behaviour*, 25(3), 15–21.

Mendelson, E. (1992) A Survey of Practice at a Regional Forensic Service: What Do Forensic Psychiatrists Do? *British Journal of Psychiatry*, 160, 769–72.

Modestin, J. (1987) Counter-Transference Reactions Contributing to Completed Suicide. *British Journal of Medical Psychology*, 60, 379–85.

Morgan, H.G. (1979) *Death Wishes? The Understanding and Management of Deliberate Self-Harm.* Chichester, Sx: Wiley.

Morgan, H.G. and Priest, P. (1984) Assessment of Suicide Risk in Psychiatric In-patients. *British Journal of Psychiatry*, 145, 467–9.

Mullen, P.E. (1993) Care and Containment in Forensic Psychiatry. *Criminal Behaviour and Mental Health*, 3, 212–25.

Myers, D.H., Leahy, A., Shoeb, H. and Ryder, J. (1990) The Patients' View of Life in a Psychiatric Hospital. *British Journal of Psychiatry*, 156, 853–60.

Neill, J.R. (1979) The Difficult Patient: Identification and Response. *Journal of Clinical Psychiatry*, 40, 209–12.

Norton, K. and Dolan, B. (1995) Acting Out and the Institutional Response. *Journal of Forensic Psychiatry*, 6(2), 317–32.

Powell, G., Caan, W. and Crowe, M. (1994) What Events Precede Violent Incidents in Psychiatric Hospitals? *British Journal of Psychiatry*, 165, 107–12.

Sandier, J., Holder, A. and Dare, C. (1970) Basic Psychoanalytic Concepts: II. The Treatment Alliance. *British Journal of Psychiatry*, 116, 555–8.

Scott, D.J. and Philip, A.E. (1985) Attitudes of Psychiatric Nurses to Treatment and Patients. *British Journal of Medical Psychology*, 58, 169–73.

The Secretary of State for Health (1992) *Report of the Committee of Inquiry into Complaints at Ashworth Hospital.* Cm. 2028. London: HMSO.

Torpy, D. and Hall, M. (1993) Violent Incidents in a Secure Unit. *Journal of Forensic Psychiatry*, 4(3), 517–44.

Valliant, G.E. (1992) The Beginning of Wisdom Is Never Calling a Patient a Borderline. *Journal of Psychotherapy Practice and Research*, 1(2), 117–34.

Watson, J.P. and Bouras, N. (1988) 'Psychiatric Ward Environments and their Effects on Patients.' In K. Granville-Grossman, ed. *Recent Advances in Clinical Psychiatry*. Edinburgh: Churchill Livingstone.

Watts, D. and Morgan, H.G. (1994) Malignant Alienation: Dangers for Patients Who Are Hard to Like. *British Journal of Psychiatry*, 164, 11–15.

Whittington, R. and Mason, T. (1995) A New Look at Seclusion: Stress, Coping and the Perception of Threat. *Journal of Forensic Psychiatry*, 6(2), 285–304.

Wieden, P. and Havens, H. (1994) Psychotherapeutic Management Techniques in the Treatment of Outpatients with Schizophrenia. *Hospital and Community Psychiatry*, 45(6), 549–55.

Winnicott, D.W. (1949) Hate in the Countertransference. *International Journal of Psychoanalysis*, 30(2), 69–74.

8

The Beginning of Wisdom is Never Calling a Patient a Borderline *or,* The Clinical Management of Immature Defenses in the Treatment of Individuals with Personality Disorders[*]

George Vaillant
1992

. . . .

Editors' reflections
Another useful way of thinking about personality disorder is to see it as a manifestation of the use of immature psychological defences. People with personality disorder lack the capacity to organise a coherent sense of self, and so cannot manage disturbing thoughts and feelings that others manage quite easily. Healthy people use a mixture of mature, neurotic and immature defences to deal with stressful situations; people with personality disorders manage stress by utilising a dysfunctional 'hand' of psychological defences. In this paper, George Vaillant emphasises how therapists working with personality disorder

[*] Originally published in *Journal of Psychotherapy Practice and Research*, 1, 2, 117–134. Reprinted with permission from the *Journal of Psychotherapy Practice and Research* © 1992 American Psychiatric Association.

need to provide a stabilising environment that acts as a 'good enough mirror' for the patient. He offers two notes of caution: first, that stigmatising and objectifying people with personality disorder is easy and unhelpful; and second, that the fact that professionals do this to service users with personality disorders rather suggests that immature defences are contagious! Vaillant's work is immensely readable and humane. We are grateful to Professor Conor Duggan for first bringing this paper to our attention.

. . . .

INTRODUCTION

The treatment of personality disorder is far less easy than the treatment of neurotic conflicts. The defenses of patients with personality disorders have become part of the warp and woof of their life histories and of their personal identities. However maladaptive their defenses may be in the eyes of the beholder, they represent homeostatic solutions to the inner problems of the user. Neurotics suffer from their defenses (which may include repression, isolation, reaction formation, and displacement) and thus welcome insight and view interpretation of their defenses as helpful. In contrast, the defenses of patients with personality disorders often only make others suffer; the owners view interpretation of their defenses as an unwarranted attack.

Nevertheless, if psychiatry, psychology, and general practice are to help their most difficult patients, the immature defenses such as projection, hypochondriasis, dissociation, fantasy, acting out, splitting, and turning against the self—the building blocks of Axis II disorders—must be understood. The appreciation of immature defenses is essential to reaching the hypochondriacal help-rejecting complainer, the wrist-cutting borderline, the injustice-collecting litigant, the devaluing eccentric, and the noncompliant sociopath—in short, the denizens of any urban emergency room on a Saturday night. However, by carelessly threatening an immature defense, a clinician can evoke enormous anxiety and depression in the patient and rupture the therapist–patient relationship. Indeed, there is the rub. Any attempts to challenge immature defenses should be mitigated by strong social supports (e.g. Alcoholics Anonymous), or else the patient's defense needs to be replaced by alternative defenses, usually from the neurotic or intermediate level. For example, fantasy can evolve into isolation; projection can evolve into reaction formation; and hypochondriasis can evolve into displacement (Vaillant, 1977).

But helping a patient alter defenses at the immature level is easier said than done. William James spoke of character as being "set in plaster"; Wilhelm Reich, one of the early therapeutic pioneers of personality disorder, spoke of "character armor"; and Anna Freud spoke of the "petrification" of defenses. The early psychodynamic investigators of character disorder (e.g., Reich, Glover, and Abraham) provided much that was of theoretical interest but little that was of practical clinical value. Advocating longer and longer psychoanalyses hardly offers a panacea to the over-worked urban social worker, parole officer, or emergency room physician.

Rather, it was as psychoanalysts entered prisons (e.g. Adler and Shapiro, 1969), public hospital inpatient units (e.g., Havens, 1986), and general hospital wards (e.g., Kahana and Bibring, 1964) that practical help was provided to our management of the immature defenses. Such help meant that the Freudian models of drive psychology and ego psychology had to be modified. The ego and drive models are particularly well adapted to the analysis of neurotic defenses, but the analysis of immature defenses requires conceptual models that focus more on object relations. In the symptomatology of personality disorder, scripts, role-relationship models (Horowitz, 1988) and internalized beloved and hated people play as crucial a part as do conflicts over forbidden desire and rage.

Each therapist–patient dyad must collaboratively develop a meaningful common language. This common language, like poetry, must lead toward a mutually understood reconstruction of the patient's inner life and of the patient's internalized relationships. Appreciation of the metaphors of immature defenses plays an important role in this reconstruction.

However, the therapy of personality disorders requires a broad, not a constricted, view of competing models of defense mechanisms. Steven Cooper (1989), a Boston psychoanalyst, describes some of these competing models succinctly: "One group of theorists, including Brenner, Kernberg, Schafer, and Kris, despite important differences in their theories, define defenses within a strictly intrapsychic context. Other theorists, such as Laplanche and Pontalis, Modell, and Kohut, emphasize that the function of some defense mechanisms is to maintain or preserve an object relation that, without it, would signify overriding anxiety" (p.866).

Cooper goes on to point out that in contrast to Anna Freud (1936), who proposed a classification of defenses according to the source of anxiety (such as the superego, the external world, or the strength of instinctual pressures), many object relations theorists have minimized drives. For example, Cooper quotes Modell (1984), as maintaining that: "Affects are the medium through which defenses against objects occur. Once affects are linked to objects, the process of instinct-defense becomes a process of defense against objects" (p.879). In his efforts to help personality disordered individuals, Kohut moved still further away from the defenses-against-drive model. Kohut (1984) maintained that the whole concept of defense-resistance is dependent on the overemphasis by classical psychoanalysis on the mechanics of mental processes to the exclusion of the patient's self-experience.

FIRST PRINCIPLES

I believe that therapists of personality-disordered patients can use help from every competent theorist they can find. Drives, people, reality, and culture are all significant. Psychoanalysis, family systems theory, cognitive therapy, and behavior modification can all play valuable roles. In this article, however, I wish to focus solely upon the clinical management of immature defenses in the treatment of individuals with personality disorders. I will begin by outlining three broad principles for enabling patients to replace immature defenses with more mature defenses: stabilizing the external environment, altering the internal environment, and controlling countertransference.

Stabilizing external environment

First, an effective way to alter a person's choice of defensive style under stress is to make his or her social milieu more predictable and supportive. That is why Kohut's theories have seemed so useful to clinicians working with personality disorders. We are all a little schizoid and paranoid when among strangers whom we fear may treat us harshly. We are all more adept at altruism, suppression, and playful sublimation when among friends who are empathic toward our pain. Thus, in the consulting room, schizoid and paranoid personalities are rarely attractive, but they respond better to our empathy and forbearance than to our confrontation or rejection. Indeed, Kohut's views on the treatment of personality disorders remind me of the old fable of the wind and the sun competing to see who can make a traveler remove his overcoat. The harder the wind blew, the more tightly the man defended himself with his overcoat. Then, it was the sun's turn; and when the sun shone down, of course, the man grew warm and cast his outer garments aside.

Similarly, the more the drive-oriented psychiatrists tug at their patients' mantle of defenses, the more they will see the immature defenses exaggerated. In contrast, the "Winnicottian" or "Kohutian" who strives empathically to be a good enough mirror or self object for the patient will find personality-disordered patients using more mature and less pathologic defenses—until the patients leave the consulting room and cloak themselves once more to meet the chilly gusts of the cold, outside world.

Altering internal environment

Second, facilitating internal as well as external safety remains a cornerstone of the treatment of personality disorders. We can also help patients abandon immature defenses by altering their internal milieu. Toxic brain syndrome makes almost anyone project. Intoxication with alcohol and unlanced abscesses of grief and anger lead to fantasy, to rage turned against the self, and to acting-out. We are all better at sublimation and reaction formation when we are not hungry, not tired, and not lonely. Often, adequate pharmacotherapy of affective spectrum disorder can ameliorate symptoms of Axis II disorders that are secondary to affective illness.

In addition, if we attempt to challenge patients' defenses, we must be sure that we have their permission. If in the course of examination we ask our patients to remove their protective clothing, we must protect them with something else. Psychopharmacology alone is rarely specific enough to provide such protection. Too often, psychiatrists forget that the brain was designed to process information and not as a series of mere chemoreceptors. The limbic system was neurobiologically designed to be comforted by friendly people and not by chemistry. Either we must offer these personality-disordered individuals ourselves—a luxury rarely available to busy doctors—or we must offer them alternative social systems and facilitate their use of more adaptive defenses.

Controlling countertransference

Third, if we are to manage our patients' immature defenses, we must manage our own countertransference. I believe that almost always the diagnosis "borderline" is a reflection more of therapists' affective rather than their intellectual response to their personality-disordered patients. That, perhaps, is why up to 90% of patients diagnosed "borderline" can also be assigned another, usually more discriminating, Axis II diagnosis (Angus and Marziali, 1988; Fyer et al., 1988); and even when carefully applied, the DSM-III-R criteria for borderline personality disorder are extremely overinclusive and lacking in specificity. For years I have demonstrated to our own residents the subjective nature of the epithet "borderline" by asking each of them to list what they considered the six most salient characteristics of the borderline. Year after year there is little consensus. As with beauty, the definition of "borderline" lies in the eye of the beholder. For, as a function of personality-disordered persons' need to establish object constancy, their immature defenses have an uncanny capacity to get under the skin of some observers. To circumvent such objectivity in working with patients who use immature defenses, it behooves the therapist to use the surgeon's favorite defense of isolation and to try to identify the patient's defense style as precisely as possible.

When I am invited to other centers as a visiting professor, I always ask to interview a "borderline". My task is to endeavor to offer an alternative, more rational diagnosis. At such clinical conferences, as an outsider, I am often impressed at how irrational the ward staff have become in the prolonged presence of their character-disordered patients' provocative behavior. Helping staff to intellectualize about the defenses of such patients allows the clinicians to appreciate the invasive, infuriating, separation/individuation-defying contagion of the immature defenses. Such intellectualization helps staff to regain the sane, calm reflection with which an outsider can approach the "biggest borderline" on someone else's inpatient unit.

If our inner worlds include relatively constant people toward whom in real life we have had relatively unambivalent feelings, then our external relationships will remain relatively assured, loving, autonomous, and well demarcated. However, the internalization of stable and loving people is not the lot of individuals with personality disorders. The interpersonal relationships of such individuals remain perpetually unstable and entangled. It is often in an effort to preserve an illusion of interpersonal constancy that individuals with personality disorders unconsciously deploy immature defenses. These image-distorting defenses permit ambivalent mental representations of other people to be conveniently "split" (into good and bad) or moved about and reapportioned. Too often, clinicians unconsciously, then, label the immature defenses of such patients as perverse or taboo; for, once touched, observers can rarely separate themselves from immature defenses completely.

Put differently, immature defenses are contagious. The contagion of immature defenses does much to account for the inhumanity of man to man that is seen throughout our criminal justice system. The hypochondriac provokes our passive-aggression, and, in the presence of an acting-out drug addict, liberals become prejudiced. When baited by their adolescent children, even the most reasonable and staid parents become hopelessly overinvolved and unreasonable. In such instances, we are hard put to distinguish "normal" countertransference and "pathologic" projective identification (Brandchaft and Stolorow, 1984). And yet the process by which our patients get under our skin is subtle; and the tumult, if noticed, seems quite mysterious to an outsider. Recently, I was fascinated to note that when I asked our residents to describe their own countertransference to their "borderline" patients, they collectively, but unwittingly, provided the DSM-III-R polythetic definition of borderline personality disorder. In short, the diagnosis "borderline" describes an

enmeshed clinical dyad in which at least the inner experience of both participants can begin to meet the criteria for the disorder.

I remember consulting on a hypochondriacal patient who had been
admitted to a general hospital for the 37th time. When I asked the medical
resident for the patient's present illness, the resident replied mysteriously, "She
was admitted for multiple stab wounds...inflicted in the emergency room." The
explanation was that the patient, a known hypochondriac—which is the internists' pejorative epithet for the "borderline"—had come in complaining of
chest pain. Unable to send the patient home, the exasperated staff tried to put in
a subclavian intravenous line on her right side. They missed the vein and tried
to insert the line on her left side and missed again. Then, furious and disgusted,
they had to admit their wounded patient.

The real moral of the story, however, was that the patient greatly benefited
from her week in the hospital. Her heart was healthy; it always had been. The
"stab wounds" were irrelevant; she had been wounded often before in the past.
But her hospitalization reduced her problem list from 20 problems to 3. What
she benefited from most was her first bath in a month, the comfort of clean
sheets, and the restoration of her internal milieu by intravenous fluids. For, in
response to her abusive home life, she had been continuously vomiting for a
week. To understand her illness it was necessary to look behind her
hypochondriacal camouflage and behind her help-rejecting reproach that
made her doctors so reflexively enraged. The true source of her pain was an
abusive spouse who was identified nowhere in her three-volume hospital
record. In her 36 prior admissions the hospital staff had been consistently
misled by this hypochondriacal patient who always insisted that her social
history was noncontributory. In their anger, the staff were only too ready to
remain blind to her real pain. Only recently have psychiatrists appreciated how
appropriate it may be to rediagnose many "borderlines" as having
post-traumatic stress disorder (Herman et al., 1989).

By necessity, the effective therapy of personality-disordered patients
requires that the therapist avoid becoming enmeshed in the patient's own issues
surrounding separation/individuation. It is well for clinicians to begin by
acknowledging what the family therapists have always known; namely, separa-
tion/individuation is a lifelong process. Just as war is too important to be left up
to the generals, individuation is too complex to be left up to toddlers. In other
words, the purpose of the immature or image-distorting defenses is to manage
internal and external object relations in adults as well as in children.

Just as neurotic mechanisms of defense (e.g. displacement, isolation, and
repression) transpose feelings, immature mechanisms (e.g. splitting, projection,
and hypochondriasis) magically maneuver both feelings and their objects. Psy-

chotherapists are no exception. Almost by definition, work with a personality-disordered patient creates a psychological "umbilical" link between patient and therapist. This psychic fusion, often unconscious, violates the ideal of a therapist who first provides the patient a neutral blank screen and then wisely interprets the patient's conflicts projected or transferred onto that screen. The technical but difficult-to-define term "projective identification" (Meissner, 1980) captures more abstractly the back-and-forth transfusions of affects and introjects that threaten to disrupt effective psychotherapy with patients afflicted by personality disorder.

By recognizing that the invasive, contagious quality of personality disorder "infects" and produces reciprocal projective identifications in the therapist, (Brandchaft and Stolorow, 1984) I am not saying that the phenomena that we associate with patients whom we label "borderline" are iatrogenic. For as Brandchaft and Stolorow (1991) warn, "conceptualizing borderline phenomena as arising in an intersubjective field is *not* equivalent to claiming that the term 'borderline' refers to an entirely iatrogenic illness" (p.1117). Rather, I am simply noting that in the presence of a patient who deploys image-distorting defenses, the therapist may unwittingly accept the patient's projections. Thus, in the blurring of ego boundaries that often accompanies the essentially dyadic process of projective identification (Goldstein, 1991), the therapist may forget that "borderlines" can be stabbed by the very hand held out to comfort them.

Countertransference in clinical practice

Inadvertent countertransference has led to four popular approaches for managing personality-disordered patients: psychopharmacology, mothering, limit-setting, and interpretation. These four approaches, if pursued too enthusiastically, are more likely to lead to disaster than to success.

First, psychopharmacology is often overused in managing difficult borderline patients. Borderline patients seek pills; they demand pills; they abuse pills; they try to kill themselves with pills; and they try to punish their therapist by taking too many or too few pills. In response, their therapists—urged on by hopeful advertising and their own frustration—try one after another of the latest pharmaceutical agents. The results at best are like playing roulette, and at worst such polypharmacy leads to iatrogenic multiple drug abuse. If one takes the long view, personality-disordered patients—in sharp contrast to patients with schizophrenia and major depressive disorder—fare better as Christian Scientists or as members of any group that provides patients a holding environment while simultaneously forbidding their use of psychopharmacological agents. By these words of caution I am not criticizing the use of carbamazepine, lithium, or low-dose neuroleptics (Cowdry and Gardner, 1988; Soloff *et al.*, 1986) to control unmanageable behavior in selected patients with personality disorders. Nor am I suggesting that antidepressants cannot play a critical role in ameliorating affective spectrum disorders (Hudson and Pope, 1990), which may present as personality disorders. Rather, I am only asking clinicians to wonder, each time they reach for their prescription pads, "Will my prescription reflect scientific pharmacotherapy or countertransference?"

A second equally dangerous response to personality-disordered patients is the impulse to be the "good-enough mother" that the patient never had. Responding to their idealized understanding of the wise techniques of Heinz Kohut and Margaret Mahler, such therapists try to mother, mirror, and love their patients. Borderline patients take the promise of mothering as seriously as they do the promise of a magic pill. Again, the results are often antitherapeutic. When you really need a mother—during August vacation, at three o'clock in the morning, and on Christmas day—would-be therapist-mothers, unlike real mothers, are never available. The patient, often an already angry and formerly abused child, takes such a seeming breach of faith by an allegedly kind clinician as a justified opportunity to bite the hand that feeds him. Therapists regard such treatment by their patients as ungrateful and respond by condemning their patients as having too much "innate aggression" or as being afflicted with "malignant narcissism." The fight is on. Instead of finding a good mother, the patient experiences another blow to self-esteem, hardly what the doctor wished to order.

This sequence of events may explain the transferential sequence of events that Gunderson and Zanarini (1987) have described as pathognomonic of a "borderline" diagnosis: "When the borderline person senses a supportive relationship with another person (or within the structured, warm 'hold' of institutional settings), he or she is likely to experience sustained dysphoria and a lack of self-satisfaction. When such a relationship is disrupted by the threat of separation or the withdrawal of reassuring nurturance, there is a shift to angry, hostile affect accompanied by highly characteristic manipulative, self-destructive actions" (p.5).

Instead of helping young adults with personality disorders to find mothers, the therapist should encourage such patients to be surrogate mothers, both to others and, equally important, to their own "inner child." Little is gained by forcing the personality-disordered person into the confining role of sick patient. Rather, self-esteem is enhanced by allowing the patient to be of appropriate help to others who are more needy. Furthermore, reaction formation and altruism are less troublesome ego defenses than acting out. In other words, pill-taking is rarely helpful for personality-disordered patients, but anybody's sense of object constancy, self-esteem, self-efficacy, and empowerment is often helped by giving pills to others. But such surrogate responsibility for others must occur within the matrix of a holding environment. Often this holding environment entails an institution; for institutions, like real mothers, remain at home during August, at 3 A.M., and on Christmas day. The 12th-stepper cares for others within the fellowship of AA; the former delinquent cares for others within the matrix of a fire department; the former narcissistic playboy, St. Francis, cares for others within the holding environment of a monastery.

Third, perceiving the need for limits in personality-disordered patients, many writers recommend a punitive, authoritarian Nurse Ratchet (from *One Flew over the Cuckoo's Nest*) approach. Once again, this approach is encouraged by the patients themselves. Many personality-disordered patients have "thrown stones at the jailhouse door" in order to obtain the limits that they feel they need. Yet to be inside a jail or a restricted psychiatric ward is as noxious for a personality-disordered patient as is too ready access to alprazolam or to the cheat of being promised, after age 21, a good mother. Instead of providing limits from above, the therapist should encourage peer support. Effective, structured social supports—whether Overeaters Anonymous, group therapy, or a Hell's Angels gang—render the patient's social world safer and thus reduce the need for maladaptive, image-distorting defenses. Besides, it is the presence of social support that distinguishes limits from punishment, a delicate but vitally important distinction. Although punishment is useless in mitigating personality disorders, limits, like scientific pharmacotherapy and holding environments, can be lifesaving. Sensitive individual psychotherapy can help to build an intrapsychic analogue to the external holding environment that is created by a receptive peer group.

Finally, a fourth popular treatment for personality disorder is insight-oriented psychotherapy. Once again, a treatment that seems promising to patient and therapist alike is often disappointing. The efforts of psychotherapists to interpret their patients' projection, splitting, and hypochondriasis may be disastrous. In response to psychoanalytic interpretation, neurotic patients are grateful and often decide to become psychotherapists themselves. In contrast, interpretation of the defenses of personality-disordered patients can make them feel disgusted, angered, or ashamed. If a therapist points out that a hypochondriac's help-rejecting complaining is defensive, the interpretation will result in the patient's accusing the therapist of being heartless, unfeeling, obtuse, and stupid. To tell another person that he or she is paranoid and prejudiced results in being called a bigot yourself. To point out to patients that they use schizoid fantasy is as comforting as explaining to them that their chief defect is loneliness. To tell someone in the middle of a tantrum that he or she is acting out is like trying to pacify a raging ocean by flogging it. In contrast, empathy, mirroring, and what Leston Havens (1986) calls "making contact" are most useful and allow the patient to shift from immature to neurotic defenses.

In other words, although immature defenses can be understood and managed, they can rarely be interpreted. Rather, the therapist should inquire about, and help patients to think through, the consequences of their actual or intended actions. The Socratic method stands the personality-disordered patient in better stead than all the good advice and dynamic interpretations in the world. Thus, the rest of this article will focus on helping the psychotherapist to manage, rather than to interpret, immature defenses.

Besides employing the Socratic method and facilitating his or her patients' discovery of peer supports, the therapist does well to empower patients toward developing more mature defenses. By this advice I mean that the therapist should help the patient evolve along a developmental continuum: for example, hypochondriasis can lead to reaction formation and then to altruism; fantasy can lead to isolation of affect and then progress to sublimation; sadistic passive-aggression can lead first to displacement and wit, and then to humor. Sigmund Freud summed the whole process up with his sexist quip: "A young whore makes an old nun" (Freud, 1905).

Put somewhat differently, patients should be supported to provide—rather than receive—the pills, the mothering, the limits, and the psychotherapy that borderlines seek. We should remember that it is not an accident that Florence Nightingale and Mary Baker Eddy were once themselves severe hypochondriacs. Nor should we forget that, in AA, a definition of a "pigeon" is "someone who came along just in time to keep their sponsor sober." We should not forget that, like a small child's mother, the physician's beeper is there to assert his or her value 24 hours a day. Lastly, more than one very gifted psychotherapist has met the criteria for personality disorder—once upon a time. Such a person's own transformation from patient to clinician was often catalyzed by his or her own individual psychotherapy—a psychotherapy that permitted projection to evolve into altruism, fantasy into sublimation, splitting into humor, and so on.

MANAGEMENT OF INDIVIDUAL DEFENSES

If we fail to recognize and to understand the immature defensive processes of our patients, we run the risk of taking these defenses personally and of condemning them. Therefore, I shall shift from discussing immature defenses collectively and examine them one at a time. Readers should translate my terms into their own language. The formulations presented below will be in the language of psychoanalytic psychiatry, but the language can be translated into principles consistent with cognitive and behavior therapies. Because the problems presented by personality disorder are ubiquitous, I shall use examples from the emergency room and from medical and psychiatric inpatient units as well as from psychotherapy. In general, I shall use the terminology for defenses popularized by the Freuds (Vaillant, 1977) but I will suggest instances where Kleinian terms like devaluation, idealization, and omnipotence could be substituted.

Although patients with personality disorders may be characterized by their most dominant or most rigid mechanism, each person usually deploys several defenses. Indeed, personality-disordered patients are often called "border-line"—if they tend to deploy a wide variety of immature defenses. Thus, in treating a patient with personality disorder, it may seem reductionistic to focus upon one or two defenses. However, sometimes in working with very provocative people, keeping it simple is helpful. Always, empathy toward immature defenses rather than countertransference is essential in creating a holding environment within the consulting room. For if the individual psychotherapist can understand the patient's defenses and avoid reactive contagion, the patient feels empathically understood and held.

Splitting

A defense mechanism commonly seen in patients with personality disorders is splitting. Instead of synthesizing and assimilating less-than-perfect past care-givers and instead of responding to important people in the current environment as they are, the patient divides ambivalently regarded people, both past and present, into good people and bad people. For example, in an inpatient setting some staff members are idealized and others are mindlessly devalued. The effect of such defensive behavior on a hospital ward or in a therapeutic group can be highly disruptive and often provokes the staff to turn against the patient. Splitting is best mastered if the staff members anticipate the process, discuss it at staff meetings as an intellectually interesting topic, and thus use the defense of isolation to reduce their own irritation.

In a psychotherapeutic setting, to dismiss the patient's split positive and negative affects as "just transference" is to miss the point. The therapist must work to create an atmosphere that is conducive to letting the patient experience simultaneously positive and negative aspects of important relationships, including the relationship with the therapist. Unconditional positive regard, safety, and firmness are necessary—all within the same session. This process necessitates a psychotherapeutic "container" analogous both to a Winnicott holding environment and to the kind of secure containment necessary to create energy from nuclear fusion. This is no easy task. Although it requires greater clarity of formulation, the task necessitates the same self-restraint and empathy that therapists use when supporting patients in acute grief. Splitting can evolve into its more mature counterparts of undoing and humor if the therapist helps the patient recall past loves as well as more recent resentments.

Fantasy

Many persons, especially eccentric, frightened persons—who are often labelled schizoid—make extensive use of the defense of fantasy. They seek solace and satisfaction within themselves by creating an imaginary life and imaginary friends. Often, such persons seem strikingly aloof. One needs to understand that such unsociability rests on a fear of intimacy. The clinician should maintain a quiet, reassuring manner with schizoid patients and convey interest in them without insisting on a reciprocal response. Recognition of their fear of closeness and respect for their eccentric ways are both useful. As trust develops, the schizoid patient may, with great trepidation, reveal a plethora of fantasies, autistic relationships, and fears of unbearable dependency, even fears of merging with the clinician. Imaginary friends should never be made fun of or even mentioned to the patient without the patient's tacit permission. The patient may vacillate between fear of clinging to the clinician and fears of fleeing through fantasy and withdrawal. Always, therapists must beware of projecting their own loneliness that the schizoid person may engender in them. They must remember to treat the schizoid character as if he or she were frightened rather than lonely.

Hypochondriasis

This mechanism of defense, also called "help-rejecting complaining," is commonly seen in patients with Axis II personality disorders—especially those with a borderline or self-defeating diagnosis. Hypochondriacs, in contrast to the usual supposition, do *not* make their complaints for simple secondary gain. A moment's reflection reveals that a hypochondriac's complaints can rarely be relieved. Often, the hypochondriac's complaint that others do not provide help conceals bereavement, loneliness, or unacceptable aggressive impulses. In other words, hypochondriasis disguises reproach and permits patients to covertly punish others through frustrating their desire to relieve the patient's own pain and discomfort. Hypochondriacs are people who bite the hands that feed them; they are not people, like conversion hysterics, who gratefully bask in the warmth of special attention. The initial response of clinicians to the hypochondriac is often guilt at their own failure to relieve suffering. This response is followed by anger and rejection on the part of the clinician, which only amplifies the patient's now vindicated reproach. Depending on the medical specialty of the caregiver being reproached, the hypochondriac may present unrelievable complaints of somatic pain or of suicidal ideation. The clinician's inadvertently angry response to this reproach may be polysurgery, or polypharmacy, or intensive psychiatric treatment followed by abrupt discharge or transfer.

Instead of trying to gratify or to diminish the hypochondriac's complaints, the care-giver should follow five rules (Brown and Vaillant, 1981). First, the clinician should acknowledge that the hypochondriac's pain or insoluble dilemma is as severe as any the interviewer has ever seen. Such amplification of the manifest complaint is an approach that, paradoxically, leads hypochondriacal patients to moderate their complaints. At last, someone has appreciated the pain of past trauma or unspeakable abuse that the hypochondriac has been unable to reveal or to emphasize. Thus, the treatment of hypochondriasis becomes an acknowledgment of the intensity and genuineness rather than the site of the pain. Instead of offering reassurance, the clinician should turn the "volume" of suffering up even further. Statements such as "I don't know how you stand it," or "It must be awful to have to endure such terrible pain," are much more hopeful than "I hope it feels a little better today." The effect of this seemingly paradoxical approach is often startling, especially when a clinician tries it and discovers, often for the first time, the beginning of a real rapport with the patient. When thus validated, the hypochondriac's painful anger can again become the patient's own responsibility.

Second, the clinician should make some symbolic effort to meet the hypochondriac's overall need for dependency, rather than attend to the specific complaint. For example, explicable complaints of abdominal pain should not be met first by reassurance and then by a covertly vindictive laparotomy. Instead, the prescription might be three days of strict bed rest, a special diet, and a careful, non-invasive physical examination of the *whole* patient. Willing offers of concern, return visits by appointment, physical therapy, and diphenhydramine rather than alprazolam are helpful. However, hypochondriacal demands—in psychiatric practice these are often suicidal threats—will increase if the patient senses a withholding of treatment or an implication that the clinician believes that pain is imaginary.

Third, instead of retaliating against the helplessness and anger that hypochondriacs engender in their caregivers, clinicians need to wonder, "Why is this patient so angry?" A careful social history may provide the answer. By including a legible psychosocial history in a prominent place in the patient's record, the clinician can remind future caregivers of the most likely source of the patient's pain. Reminding future clinicians that the patient is a survivor of Buchenwald or a victim of child abuse may be more useful than providing a chart full of negative laboratory results or of psychodynamic ruminations about the last two weeks of "borderline" inpatient behavior.

Fourth, as the clinician plays detective, he or she should never regard misleading information as lying. Most hypochondriacal misinformation is as innocent and as unconscious as that of a patient with coronary disease who complains of terrible arm pain. The hypochondriacal complaint is, after all, an effort to get the doctor's attention, to validate past trauma, and to displace rage rather than an effort to obtain secondary gain or a quick fix. The need of Coleridge's "Ancient Mariner" to repeat his tale of woe provides an analogy. In acknowledging and validating past unspeakable trauma, the therapist will ultimately serve the so-called borderline, who may in fact suffer from post-traumatic stress disorder (Herman *et al.*, 1989) far better than if the therapist were to maintain too close an adherence to the theories of Mahler and Melanie Klein. Validation of past trauma is essential to the creation of a stable sense of self.

Finally, in caring for a hypochondriacal patient perhaps the most useful technique is to use the metaphor inherent in the patient's pain to link physical or self-abusive compliant to affect. A hypochondriacal patient who complains of chest pain, and who is unreassured by a normal ECG, may be comforted if the clinician says, "One thing is sure; the pain in your heart is real." Or when a patient provocatively mentions his suicidal ideation yet again, the caregiver can respond with: "I can see that things have been terribly painful for you; you must be furious that others have helped so little." In both cases the clinician, by responding with metaphor, not logic, opens the way for a broader consideration of life's pain.

These five principles permit a useful modification of the clinician's own need for omnipotence. Clinicians must become able to accept that they are not going to cure the hypochondriacal patient, just as they accept that they are not able to cure a mourner after a funeral. Rather, our task with hypochondriasis, as with the other immature defenses, is to decipher it so that we may remain sensitive to the patient's pain, not so that we can abolish it.

Many patients who use fantasy and hypochondriasis are pejoratively labelled "narcissistic." This is because both fearfulness and poor self-esteem are shored up by schizoid or hypochondriacal pretence of omnipotence. To the casual observer and to the unempathic clinician, such self-centered behavior may be erroneously labelled vanity, grandiosity, and entitlement. An effective way of surmounting the pejorative connotations of the term "narcissism" is to translate that multi-syllabic epithet into the simpler and more empathic phrase "in pain."

Patients who use splitting, fantasy, and hypochondriasis may also be unusually critical of (i.e. devalue) the clinician. Some patients may even suggest that a therapist pay for the privilege of caring for them. In response, the therapist may become defensive, contemptuous, or rejecting. Nobody likes being belittled. Clinical progress is facilitated if, instead of belittling patients or defending themselves, clinicians understand that the Kleinian defense of devaluation is a less mature cousin of the Freudian defense of undoing. What this means is that such patients are contemptuous of their clinicians precisely because the patient also feels reluctantly loving toward or admiring of them. The paradoxical contempt and envy induced by perceiving one's therapist as lovable can only be transformed into gratitude by sustained Rogerian unconditional positive regard and by Kohutian mirroring. No easy task.

Projection

Another defense commonly encountered in patients with personality disorders is projection. Excessive fault-finding and undue sensitivity to criticism on the patient's part may seem to the observer to be prejudiced, injustice-collecting projection. But projection, however blatant, should not be met by interpretation, defensiveness, or argument. There is usually a grain of truth in most projection! Instead, even minor mistakes on the part of the clinician and the possibility of future difficulties should be frankly acknowledged. The epithet "paranoid" should be replaced with the more empathic "hypervigilant." Strict honesty, real concern for the patient's rights, and maintaining the same formal, although concerned, distance as one would with a patient using fantasy are helpful. Confrontation guarantees a lasting enemy and an early termination of the interview. Therapists need not agree with their patients' injustice-collecting; instead, they should ask respectfully whether they can agree to disagree.

The technique of counterprojection (Havens, 1986) is especially helpful. In that technique, the clinician acknowledges and gives paranoid patients full credit for their feelings and for their perceptions. Further, the clinician neither disputes the patient's complaints nor reinforces them; rather, he or she acknowledges that the world that the paranoid describes is imaginable.

There are several components to counterprojection. First, the clinician aligns him or herself beside, not opposite, the patient. Eye contact and confrontation are avoided and replaced with the interactive mode of a traveling companion who is trying to view the world from a similar vantage point. Both clinician and patient look out of the same bus window, as it were.

Second, empathic counterprojective statements must encompass, without necessarily agreeing with, the patients' distress. Thus, Havens (1986) uses the example of a patient stubbing his toe, to which the therapist responds, "That damned old chair!" rather than "That must have hurt."

Third, the point of counterprojection is not to agree with the patient, but only to get out of the way. Thus, the therapist would not say, "The doctors in this hospital are sadists," but "It must seem as if the doctors here were trying to make you suffer." In so doing, the clinician distances him or herself from the patient's tormentors. The interviewer can then talk about the patient's real motives and feelings, even though they are initially misattributed to someone else.

Fourth, unlike the case with hypochondriasis, where metaphorical speech is important, with paranoid patients precise speech is helpful. In addition, a statement—what Havens (1986) calls "making marks"—is more revealing and less annoying than a question. Whereas the interrogatory "When were you born?" will meet with a rebuff, the statement "I expect that you are a Gemini (or born in June)" will elicit "No, I was born in September."

The clinician must remember that trust and tolerance of intimacy are troubled areas for paranoid patients. Courtesy, honesty, and respect are the cardinal rules for the treatment of any such patient. If the clinician is accused of some actual inconsistency or fault, such as lateness for an appointment, an honest apology serves better than a defensive explanation or an analytic "Mmm?"

Individual psychotherapy requires a professional and not overly warm style on the therapist's part, and argument over trustworthiness is futile. For example, consider the following dialogue:

PATIENT: I am sure this room is bugged.

THERAPIST: To the best of my knowledge it is not.

PATIENT: I could not trust a psychiatrist who bugs his office.

THERAPIST: Any sensible person would mistrust a psychiatrist who bugged his office. I expect it's a waste of time, but, if you wish, you can look for bugs. On the other hand, you may have some other topics you would rather talk about.

Too zealous a use of interpretation—especially interpretation concerning deep feelings of dependency, sexual concerns, and wishes for intimacy—significantly increases the patient's mistrust. Clinicians can often address the concerns concealed behind projection if they wait until the patient brings up these concerns in a displaced manner; for with maturation, projection evolves naturally into displacement and reaction formation.

At times, the behavior of paranoid patients becomes so threatening that it is important to control or set limits on it. Delusional accusations must be dealt with realistically but gently and without humiliating the patient. When disorganized by high levels of anxiety, paranoid patients can be reassured by the clinician's involving security personnel. However, it is profoundly frightening for paranoid patients to feel that those trying to help them are weak and helpless. Therefore, a clinician should never threaten to take over control unless willing and able to do so.

Acting out

Antisocial personalities are especially prone to use acting out. Acting out represents the direct expression through action of an unconscious wish or conflict in order to avoid being conscious of either the idea or the affect that accompanies it. Tantrums, apparently motiveless assaults, child abuse, and pleasureless promiscuity are common examples. To the observer, acting out often appears to be unaccompanied by guilt, but acting out is not that simple. As with conversion hysteria and its accompanying *belle indifference*, anxiety and pain also exist behind the cool indifference of acting out. In responding to such behavior, the clinician should remember the maxim "Nothing human is alien to me."

Glover (1960) has said of the sociopath: "In addition to his incapacity to form deep personal attachments and his penchant to cause suffering to those who are attached to him, the psychopath is essentially a non-conformist, who in his reaction to society combines hostility with a sense of grievance" (p.128). But the "incapacity" of sociopaths to form attachments represents defensive process, not inability. Close relationships arouse anxiety in them. Terrified of their own dependency, of their very real "grievances," and of their fantasies of mutual destruction, sociopaths either flee relationships or destroy them.

In trying to treat the antisocial personality, the clinician must remember that these persons uniformly lacked benevolent, sustained relationships with their parents. They are afraid of intimacy and of assuming responsibility for it. They cannot believe that others can tolerate their anxiety, and they devoutly fear responsibility for achieving success by open competition. They can neither identify with authority figures nor accept their criticism, and they resent any thwarting of their actions, even when such intervention is clearly in their interest. Their consciences are too rigid, not too lenient; and so, rather than experience their own punitive self-judgment, they reject all moral standards and ideals. The eye-for-an-eye morality of street gangs, of terrorist organizations, and of the jailhouse subculture make Calvinist morality seem libertine by comparison.

Bowlby (1963) has suggested that mourning in childhood is characterized by a persistent and unconscious yearning to recover the lost object. The persistent crime and multiple drug abuse of the chronic user of acting out often represents a similar quest. Bowlby tells us that in lieu of depression, bereaved children, like sociopaths, exhibit intense and persistent anger that is expressed as reproach toward various objects, including the self. However, Bowlby notes that such anger, if misunderstood, seems often pointless enough to the outsider. Finally, sociopaths, like children, often employ secret anodynes to make loss unreal and overt grief unnecessary. Their need for secrecy is based on the fact that "to confess to another belief that the loved object is still alive is plainly to court the danger of disillusion" (p.519). These defensive maneuvers, then, serve to hide the child's and the sociopath's depression from our psychiatric view. Persistent, seemingly mindless delinquencies make symbolic sense if interpreted dynamically—as one might interpret misbehavior in a dream or in a child's play therapy. In short, I believe that the incomprehensible behavior of acting out is a product of a well-defended ego and of a strict, albeit primitive, conscience. Cleckley (1941) is wrong. Acting out is no mere "mask of sanity," but it is often a mask to grief (Vaillant, 1975).

Unlike conversion hysteria, however, acting out must be controlled as rapidly as possible. First, prolonged acting out is frightening to patient and staff alike. Faced with acting out—either aggressive or sexual—in an interview situation, the clinician must recognize that the patient has lost control. Anything that the clinician says will probably be misheard, and getting the patient's attention is of paramount importance. Depending on how threatened the clinician feels, the clinician's response can be, "You have acted in this manner because you can't pull that feeling up into your head," or, "How can I help you if you keep on screaming?" Or if the clinician feels that the patient's loss of control is escalating, he or she can respond, "If you continue screaming, I'll leave." Or, if physical violence genuinely seems a possibility, the clinician may simply leave and ask for help, including the police. Invariably, acting out begets fear in the observer, and nobody working with psychiatric patients should bear this fear alone.

Second, once acting out is no longer possible, the conflict behind the defense may be accessible. This is another reason that the clinician must find some way of limiting the patient's frightening but ultimately self-defeating behavior. To overcome the patient's fear of intimacy, the clinician must frustrate the patient's wish to run from tenderness and from the honest pain of human encounter. In doing so, the clinician faces the challenge of differentiating control from punishment and of differentiating help and confrontation from social isolation and retribution. Successful models of the controlling, helping, confrontational environment include halfway-house residences enforced by probation, "addiction" to methadone clinics, and the kind of therapeutic community behind bars that was devised for sociopaths at Utah State Hospital (Kiger, 1967) and that was formerly achieved at the Patuxent Institute in Jessup, Maryland, and the Herstevester in Denmark. If those who use acting out are prevented from flight or tantrum, or if they are approached by understanding peers, instead of appearing incorrigible, inhuman, unfeeling, guiltless, and unable to learn from experience, they become only too human.

Third, chronic users of acting out should be encouraged to find alternative defense mechanisms. Play is always preferable to war. Displacement is the more mature cousin of acting out. As with a young child, the clinician should not just tell an antisocial person to stop doing something, but should point the patient toward an affectively exciting alternative. Acting out needs to be redirected, not forbidden.

Finally, once those who have antisocial personalities feel that they are among peers, they often find the motivation for change that they had lacked in other settings. Perhaps that is the reason that self-help groups have often been more effective in alleviating these disorders than have jails and psychiatric hospitals.

Turning against the self

A commonly seen mechanism in patients with personality disorders is turning anger against the self. In military psychiatry and DSM-III-R, such behavior is called passive-aggressive; in psychoanalytic terminology such behavior is most often described as masochism. "Long-suffering" and "self-sacrificing" are more empathic adjectives than "masochistic," which implies that the patient suffers because it is fun. The defense of turning against the self includes failure, procrastination, silly or provocative behavior, and self-demeaning clowning, as well as more frankly self-destructive behavior. The hostility in passive aggression and masochism, however, is never entirely concealed. Indeed, behaviors like wrist-cutting engender such anger in others that they feel that they themselves have been assaulted; thus, they come to view the wrist-slasher as a sadist, not a masochist. In Massachusetts, attempted suicide used to be classified as a felony.

The best way to deal with turning against the self is by helping the patient to ventilate anger and to direct his or her assertiveness outward rather than against the self. It is important to treat the suicidal gestures of passive-aggressive patients as one would any covert expression of anger and not as one would treat grief or primary depression. Antidepressant medications should be prescribed only when clinical indications are pressing and only when the possibility of overdose has been seriously weighed.

However, just as it is seldom wise to respond to angry suicidal patients as though they were simply depressed, it is seldom wise to isolate such patients in seclusion rooms for their angry gestures. As in the management of hypochondriasis, the therapist's task is to help patients acknowledge their anger, not to act out the patients' anger for them. The relief of tension that some patients obtain from repeatedly cutting or burning themselves should be accepted as matter-of-factly by the clinician as the clinician would tolerate equally dangerous two-pack-a-day smoking in a colleague. Rather than treating self-inflicted cigarette burns as perverse or dangerous, staff members should say gently, "I wonder if there's some other way you could make yourself feel better. Can you put what you are feeling into words?" The clinician must continually point out the probable consequences of passive-aggressive behavior as they occur. Questions such as, "What do you really want for yourself?" may help to change the patient's behavior more than would a corrective interpretation or, as is all too common, instituting retaliatory suicidal restrictions.

Therapeutic techniques that help channel the patient's anger away from passive resistance and into more productive expression are very helpful. One means is to recognize that passive aggression can be channelled into displacement and humor. Instead of self-deprecatory clowning and sadistic hotfoots, wit, parody, caricature, even "guerrilla theatre" offer more acceptable ways of redirecting anger formerly turned against the self.

Behavioral therapy techniques, such as assertiveness training and the explicit setting of limits, are often useful. If stubborn, passive-aggressive patients are reluctant to help themselves, it is sometimes useful to take a time-out. Leaving the room or postponing the next appointment breaks the pattern of struggle and underscores the point that passive-aggressive struggles result in less rather than more attention. After a short time-out, the interviewer, too, is able to continue the relationship in a less angry and covertly sadistic manner (Perry and Flannery, 1989).

Recovery may be usefully presented to the long-suffering patient as a special additional task. Sometimes long-suffering, self-sacrificing patients are more able to cooperate in a medical regimen because of their readiness to add to the burdens that they carry rather than for the sake of benefits that might accrue to themselves. In every interaction with self-defeating patients, however, it is important to avoid humiliating comments about foolish, inexplicable behavior. Nobody's pride is easier to wound than that of a person who continually shoots him or herself in the foot.

Dissociation/neurotic denial

This defense (or these defenses) involves the patient's replacing unpleasant affects with pleasant ones. In its most extreme form, dissociation is manifested by multiple personality disorder. In childhood and for short periods in adult life, such denial can serve to mitigate an otherwise unbearable affect. For example, if honest self-awareness and expression repeatedly brought down abuse from caretakers, dissociation allows abused children to remain separated from their emotional experience; but, of course, dissociation does not make problems disappear. Whereas the previously mentioned defenses tend to contaminate the intersubjective field by eliciting negative affects in the therapists, the danger of dissociation within the intersubjective field is countertransferential seduction. Dependent longing and unacknowledged grief are misperceived as sexual excitement or counterphobic exuberance.

Persons using dissociation often proclaim that they feel fine, although their underlying anxiety, depression, or resentment may be obvious to others. Because their troubling affects, impulses, and wishes are disavowed and actively pushed out of consciousness, users of dissociation have a tendency to feel accused and devalued if anyone points out their troubles. They are often seen as dramatizing, theatrical, and emotionally shallow. While they may often be labelled correctly as "histrionic" personalities, "captivating" is a less pejorative adjective. Their behavior is reminiscent of the stunts of anxious adolescents who, to erase anxiety, carelessly expose themselves to exciting danger. To accept such patients as enthralling and enthralled is to become blind to their pain and neediness, but to confront them with their vulnerabilities and defects is to make them more defensive still.

Because patients who use dissociation seek appreciation of their attractiveness and courage and because they need some expression of prohibited impulses, the clinician should not be too reserved—only calm and firm. Reframing vulnerabilities as opportunities or potential strengths is often more effective than confronting such patients with their defects. Rather than lecture a "macho" coronary care patient, "Mr. Jones, you have had a very severe heart attack. You may die if you do not follow unit regulations," a better approach may be, "Mr. Jones, it takes real guts to put up with inactivity and the CCU routines, but remember, every day that you can tough out the pain of bed rest, your heart is getting stronger."

Such patients are often imaginative, if inadvertent, liars, but they benefit from having a chance to ventilate their own anxieties. In the process of free association they often "remember" what they "forgot", and through psychotherapy their self-serving lies can revolve into the acknowledgment of painful truths. Therefore, dissociation and neurotic denial are best dealt with if the clinician uses displacement and talks with the patient about the same affective issue but in a less threatening context. Empathizing with the denied affect, without directly confronting patients with the facts, may allow them to reintroduce the original painful topic themselves.

CONCLUSION

Let me close this discussion of immature defenses with four final suggestions on how to use an understanding of these defenses in individual psychotherapy.

First, defenses, especially immature (i.e. image-distorting) defenses, occur in a rich and complex interpersonal, intersubjective context. Such defenses encompass real past relationships and present, if primitive, transferences, as well as the realities of the current doctor–patient relationship. The simplified techniques outlined above for managing these defenses are offered only as suggestions and guides to the complexities of individual psychotherapy. Like all suggestions for managing intimate and intense interpersonal relationships, such suggestions must be carried out with sensitivity to context and mutuality.

Second, the greater the variety of immature defenses that patients deploy, the more likely they are to be labelled "borderline." I believe, therefore, that using that term will always obscure differential diagnosis. Worse yet, such name-calling leads to perceiving such patients' defenses as attacks on the clinician. If readers believe that they can use the epithet "borderline" while maintaining clinical objectivity, let me invite them to try the experiment of imagining that they found themselves described in their own therapist's notes as a "borderline." Instead of name-calling, therapists should always find something to admire in their patients' attempts to master past pain. In their formulations, if not in their diagnoses, therapists need to reframe the Axis II labels so that paranoid becomes "hypervigilant," narcissistic becomes "in pain," hysterical becomes "captivating," masochistic becomes "long-suffering," schizoid becomes "independent," and borderline becomes "post-traumatic stress disorder"—or "that patient who sure knows how to push my buttons."

Third, therapists should also always find something to admire in their patients' attempts to change and grow. Taking genuine pleasure in a patient's attempts to try out new, more adaptive behaviors is very rewarding for patient and clinician alike. Therapists must remember that the personality disorders are dynamic. Like adolescents, patients with personality disorders outgrow their difficulties with a little help from time and their friends. Paranoids can become reformers; hypochondriacs can become healers; and sociopaths can become enforcers of the law. In short, the therapy of personality disorder always proceeds more smoothly if we can remember our own recovery from adolescence.

However, no defense can be abruptly altered or abandoned without an acceptable substitute. For example, abstinence from drugs is achieved through a process analogous to mourning: slowly the depended-upon substance is replaced with other loves. In similar fashion, successful treatment of personality disorder demands that the clinician try to help the patient develop a substitute for each defense.

Finally, in treating personality disorder we have to modify the conventional doctor–patient model. One-to-one therapeutic relationships by themselves are rarely sufficient to change severe personality disorder. Immature defenses repel, wound, and overwhelm the efforts of individuals; burnout is common. Only an extended family or self-help group can withstand such assault. In addition, the "borderline" needs to absorb more of other people than one person, no matter how loving, can ever provide. Nor can we look for help from drugs; there is no drug that can teach us Chinese or that can replace parents who were abusive or inconsistent throughout our childhoods.

Like adolescents, individuals with personality disorders need opportunities to internalize fresh role models and to make peace with the imperfect familial figures who are already within. A clinician, even five times a week, is not enough to satisfy an orphan. Especially at the start of the recovery process, only a church, a self-help residential treatment, or addicting drugs provide relief for a borderline's pain; all three provide an external holding environment 24 hours a day. On the other hand, individual psychotherapy, with its capacity to provide self objects and mirroring, may be more effective in modifying and enhancing those psychic structures that maintain an internal holding environment.

In other words, some form of self-help group is a useful adjunct to psychotherapy. To begin with, personality-disordered individuals, like the rest of us, need to find groups to which they can belong with pride. They often know only too well that they have harmed others; but they can meaningfully identify only with people who feel as guilty as themselves. They can abandon their defenses against grief only in the presence of people equally bereaved. Only acceptance by peers or a "higher power" can circumvent their profound fear of being pitied. Only acceptance by "recovered" peers can restore their defective self-esteem. A therapist's love is not enough.

There is another reason for combining peer groups with one-on-one therapy. Intensive individual psychotherapy seems most useful for people who (like many clinicians) have had too much parenting and for people who have learned from society not wisely but too well. In contrast, patients with personality disorders have experienced inconsistent or too little parenting. Because of defects in genes, socialization, and maturation, personality-disordered individuals have had difficulty learning what society wished to teach them. Thus, individuals with personality disorder often need care that is very similar to the care required by adolescents. Indeed, adolescents do not need therapy at all; they need a social group that offers them time, space, and safety to internalize the valuable facets of their parents and their society and to extrude the chaff. They need mentors and loves in order to catalyze the developmental transmutation whereby adolescent envy becomes adult gratitude. Object constancy—as defined by Kernberg (1968) not Piaget—is an essential ingredient of maturity; and object constancy is lacking both in adolescents and in personality disorder. The task of therapy for personality-disordered individuals, then, is to create such object constancy. For adults, groups and institutions sometimes provide this constancy and the opportunities for fresh identifications more consistently than can a single individual a few hours a week. At the same time, individual psychotherapy can play a vital role in the treatment of personality disorder. It is easier to walk with two crutches than with one.

SUMMARY

In individual psychotherapy of personality disorders, patients' uses of the less mature ego mechanisms of defense can detrimentally affect the intersubjective field. The diagnostic epithet "borderline" often reflects unconscious countertransference more than it does diagnostic precision. Psychotherapists can avoid the deleterious effects of such countertransference by being attentive to the ways their patients' defensive styles affect the therapeutic dyad and by learning to collaborate with self-help groups. The author discusses strategies for managing in individual psychotherapy seven immature or image-distorting defense mechanisms: splitting, schizoid fantasy, hypochondriasis, projection, turning against the self, acting out, and neurotic denial.

This article owes much to my sustained collaboration with J. Christopher Perry, M.D., and Leigh McCullough, Ph.D., and to three anonymous reviewers. The work was supported by research grants K05MH00364, MH39799 and MH42248, National Institute of Mental Health.

REFERENCES

Adler, C. and Shapiro, L.N. (1969) 'Psychotherapy with prisoners.' In J. Masserman, (ed.) *Current Psychiatric Therapies 1*, vol 9. New York: Grune and Stratton. p.99–105.

Angus, L.E. and Marziali, E. (1988) A comparison of three measures for the diagnosis of borderline personality disorder. *American Journal of Psychiatry,* 145, 1453–1454.

Bowlby,J. (1963) Pathological mourning and childhood mourning. *Journal of the American Psychoanalytic Association,* 11, 500–541.

Brandchaft, B. and Stolorow, R. (1984) 'The borderline concept: Pathological character or iatrogenic myth.' In J. Lichtenberg, M. Bernstein and D. Silver, (eds) *Empathy, vol 2.* Hillsdale, NJ: Analytic Press. p.333–357.

Brandchaft, B. and Stolorow, R.D. (1991) The borderline concept. *Journal of the American Psychoanalytic Association,* 38, 1117–1119.

Brown, H.N. and Vaillant, G.E (1981) Hypochondriasis. *Archives of Internal Medicine,* 141, 723–726.

Cleckley, H. (1941) *The Mask of Sanity.* St. Louis, MO: CV Mosby.

Cooper, S. (1989) Recent contributions to the theory of defense mechanisms: A comparative view. *Journal of the American Psychoanalytic Association,* 37, 865–893.

Cowdry, R.W. and Gardner, D.L. (1988) Pharmacotherapy of borderline personality disorder. *Archives of General Psychiatry,* 45, 113–119.

Freud, A. (1936) *The Ego and the Mechanisms of Defense.* London: Hogarth Press.

Freud, S. (1905) 'Three essays on the theory of sexuality.' In J. Strachey, (ed.) (1962) *The Standard Edition of the Complete Psychological Works of Sigmund Freud, vol 7.* London: Hogarth Press. p.130–24.

Fyer, M.R., Frances, A.J., Sullivan, T. *et al.* (1988) Comorbidity of borderline personality disorder. *Archives of General Psychiatry,* 45, 348–352.

Glover, E. (1960) *The Roots of Crime.* New York: International Universities Press.

Goldstein, W.N. (1991) Clarification of projective identification. *American Journal of Psychiatry,* 148, 153–162.

Gunderson, J.G. and Zanarini, M.C. (1987) Current overview of the borderline diagnosis. *Journal of Clinical Psychiatry,* 48[8, Suppl]:5–11.

Havens, L. (1986) *Making Contact.* Cambridge, MA: Harvard University Press.

Herman, J.L., Perry, J.C., van der Kolk, B.A. (1989) Childhood trauma in borderline personality disorder. *American Journal of Psychiatry,* 146, 490–495.

Horowitz, M.J. (1988) *Introduction to Psychodynamics.* New York: Basic Books.

Hudson, J.I. and Pope, H.G. (1990) Affective spectrum disorder: Does antidepressant response identify a family of disorders with a common pathophysiology? *American Journal of Psychiatry,* 147, 552–574.

Kahana, R.J. and Bibring, C.L. (1964) 'Personality types in medical management.' In N. Zinberg, (ed.) *Psychiatry and Medical Practice in a General Hospital.* New York: International Universities Press. p.108–123.

Kernberg, O. (1968) The treatment of patients with borderline personality organization. *International Journal of Psychoanalysis,* 49, 600–619.

Kiger, R. (1967) Treatment of the psychopath in the therapeutic community. *Hospital and Community Psychiatry,* 18,191–196.

Kohut, H. (1984) *How Does Analysis Cure?* Chicago: University of Chicago Press.

Meissner, W. (1980) A note on projective identification. *Journal of the American Psychoanalytic Association,* 28, 43–67.

Modell, A. (1984) *Psychoanalysis in a New Context.* New York: International Universities Press.

Perry, J.C. and Flannery, R. (1989) 'Dependent personality disorder.' In T.B. Karasu, (ed.) *Treatment of Psychiatric Disorders, Vol 3.* Washington, DC: American Psychiatric Press, pp.2762–2770.

Perry, J.C. and Vaillant, G.E. (1988) 'Personality disorders.' In H. Kaplan and B. Sadock, (eds) *Comprehensive Textbook of Psychiatry.* Baltimore: Williams and Wilkins.

Soloff, P.H., Anselm, G., Swami, N.S. *et al.* (1986) Progress in pharmacotherapy of borderline disorders. *Archives of General Psychiatry,* 43, 691–697.

Vaillant, G.E. (1975) Sociopathy as a human process. *Archives of General Psychiatry,* 32, 179–189.

Vaillant, G.E. (1977) *Adaptation to Life.* Boston: Little, Brown.

9

Psychiatric Staff as Attachment Figures: Understanding Management Problems in Psychiatric Services in the Light of Attachment Theory*

Gwen Adshead

1998

. . . .

Editors' reflections

Attachment theory has become an incredibly useful theoretical and practical framework for understanding difficult and complex service users and their problems. It argues that psychological development and functioning are affected by our earliest attachments to care-givers. Failed or pathological attachment in childhood may give rise to repetition of maladaptive attachment patterns in adulthood. If this is the case, then we should expect service users with histories of failed or toxic attachments to carers, to really struggle when they meet professional carers. Either they will repeat a previous negative attachment pattern that they had with their early care-givers; or they may resist making any therapeutic attachments at all, and be hostile towards carers. What carers need to do is to try to make themselves psychologically 'secure', to try to prevent a repeat of the past.

. . . .

* Originally published in *British Journal of Psychiatry*, 172, 64–69. © 1998 The Royal College of Psychiatrists.

INTRODUCTION

Attachment theory has been a powerful influence on child psychiatry, psycho-therapy, and psychotherapy research. Bowlby (1988) first postulated that attachment to others has an ethological basis, producing behaviours which are driven by a need for relationships, rather than food or sex. This paper will focus on the implications of attachment theory for general practice. I will discuss whether relationships between general psychiatric patients and mental health care professionals in general psychiatric environments could be characterised as 'attachment' relationships. An understanding of therapeutic relationships within psychiatric services, based on attachment theory, may offer a new per-spective on management and behavioural problems that occur in clinical practice.

ATTACHMENT BEHAVIOUR AND THEORY

Attachment theory holds that humans are essentially social animals who need relationships for survival, and whose first relationships with parental figures have unique characteristics (Bowlby, 1988). Attachment behaviour is any form of behaviour that results in a person attaining or maintaining proximity to an 'attachment figure', usually a care-giver. Such behaviour is most obvious when people are frightened, fatigued or sick, and is assuaged by comforting and care-giving (Bowlby, 1979). It can be seen throughout the life cycle, especially in emergencies, and its biological function appears to be the protection of the developing and vulnerable organism.

Weiss (1991) suggests that relationships can only be properly called attach-ments if they display specific attachment properties, including proximity-seeking, elicitation by threat, and the use of attachments as a secure base. To say that a person is attached to, or has an attachment to another, is to say that they are strongly disposed to seek proximity to and contact with that individual, and to do so especially under certain specified conditions. Both the quality and the strength of the attachment are important.

In psychological terms, secure attachment relationships allow the develop-ing individual to construct 'internal working models', of himself and others, based on the interaction between himself and the attachment figure, which become established as internal cognitive structures (Main et al., 1985). These structures provide a framework for cognitive processing of perceptions, events and relationships, and the development of belief systems and cognitive schemata. Kraemer (1992) proposes a neurophysiological basis for such cognitive models.

Bowlby's theory proposes that attachment behaviour functions as a kind of homeostatic mechanism for modulating anxiety. Increasing anxiety and arousal increases attachment behaviour; thus, the goal of attachment behaviour can be seen as helping the individual to modulate their anxiety and arousal. Their own chosen attachment figure is best, but failing this, any attachment figure will do. A cold, unhelpful figure is likely to be better than nothing at all.

PSYCHOLOGICAL EFFECTS OF INSECURE ATTACHMENT

Most of the early research on attachment in non-human primates studied the effects of failed attachment, usually as a result of early separation. Failed attachment resulted in disturbances of social behaviour, such as sexual behaviour and grooming.

In humans, the nature and quality of attachment has been studied in infants by looking at infant behaviour in an unfamiliar situation (Ainsworth *et al.*, 1978). Three main categories of insecure attachment in children are described as avoidant, ambivalent and disorganised. In adults, security of attachment style is assessed by linguistic analysis of memories of parenting, recalled in a semi-structured interview (Adult Attachment Interview (AAI); Main and Goldwyn, 1989). Three insecure attachment styles have been described: dismissing, preoccupied and unresolved following trauma or loss.

Could early insecurity of attachment be a risk factor, predisposing factor or causative agent of later psychiatric disorder? Most developmental researchers would argue for an interactional model of development. Rutter (1995) suggests that failure of early attachment may be a risk factor for later adult psychiatric disorder, by interacting with other vulnerability and resilience factors to increase or decrease the risk of psychiatric disorder in adulthood. If psychiatric disorder were understood as a failure of the organism to manage neuro-physiological and psychological homeostasis, then it would be plausible to argue that probably the majority of those with psychiatric disorders will have histories of failed or pathological attachments, even though only a minority of those individuals with failed or pathological attachments will develop psychiatric disorder.

INSECURE ATTACHMENT AND PSYCHIATRIC DIAGNOSES

Most research has been retrospective rather than prospective, and has studied attachment histories in vulnerable subjects. For example, depression in adulthood is associated with the loss of an attachment figure in early life

(Brown and Harris, 1978), and hostility from parents (Parker, 1983). Disturbances of attachment have been found in patients with major psychiatric illnesses, such as schizophrenia or manic-depressive illness (Dozier, 1990) and other disorders, such as pathological bereavement reactions (Parkes, 1991). A recent meta-analysis found that insecure attachments were over-represented in clinical populations (van Ijzendoorn and Bakermans Kranenburg, 1996).

Abuse, attachment and personality disorder

One particular area of childhood experience which might be relevant to attachment history is that of abuse and neglect. If abuse-related insecurity of attachment were a risk factor for psychiatric disorder, then one might expect to see an over-representation of abused adults in psychiatric populations. Some studies confirm this (for review see Mullen *et al.*, 1993). Mullen *et al.* found that a history of abuse in childhood significantly increased risk of later adult psychiatric disorder.

Attachment history is likely to be relevant to the study and treatment of personality disorders, where pathological interpersonal relationships are a key diagnostic feature. High rates of both sexual and physical abuse by parents have been found in populations of women diagnosed as suffering from borderline personality disorder (BPD) (Ogata *et al.*, 1990), and women who deliberately harm themselves (Van der Kolk *et al.*, 1991). Patrick *et al.*, (1994) compared security of attachment in BPD patients with a matched group of patients with depression, using the AAI. They found increased rates of insecure attachment in the BPD group. Repetition in adulthood of childhood attachment patterns is most likely to be replicated in the context of dependency relationships, such as with their own children (Main *et al.*, 1985); which may be relevant in the aetiology of child-abusing behaviour, such as Munchausen's syndrome by proxy.

There may be an interesting connection between insecurity of attachment, as a result of childhood trauma, and post-traumatic stress disorders. In adults, the psychodynamic effects of external disasters on the internal world include disturbance of internal homeostasis, and a massive challenge to neurotic defences against fears of abandonment (Garland, 1991). Reactions to extreme threats to security, with concomitant levels of internal anxiety, are likely to be modified by cognitive schemata (*cf.* internal working models). Adults' perception of threat, and risk of post-traumatic stress disorder, may depend on patterns of attachment and responses to trauma in early life (Bremner *et al.*, 1993). It is possible that attachment-based research could provide an empirical base for Freud's concept of repetition-compulsion as a means of mastering trauma.

Therefore, it is reasonable to anticipate that patients with a history of failed or insecure attachment are likely to be commonly present on psychiatric wards. These are likely to be individuals whose internal cognitive models make it difficult for them to manage stressors, and who may have developed maladaptive behavioural strategies in response to either internal or external stressors.

Psychiatric illness and attachment behaviour

Do relationships between psychiatric patients and mental health care professionals show the qualities of attachment relationships? Illness generally stimulates attachment behaviour and proximity-seeking to health care professionals because it is anxiety provoking, and because patients are rendered vulnerable by their illness (Bowlby, 1979). Psychiatric illness is likely to be a particularly potent stimulator of attachment behaviour because of the threat to internal as well as external safety.

The principal functions of any attachment figure are to provide a secure base and to modulate anxiety. In a health care setting, both functions are achieved by an interactional process to which both the individual and the health care professional contribute. Professional carers may be seen as providing the patient with a temporary attachment figure. Attachment figures stimulate secure attachment in dependants by spending time in 'active reciprocal interaction' (Rutter, 1988); this could be a description of various ward-based therapeutic activities. Secure attachment will be facilitated by accuracy, sensitivity and appropriate responses to distress; neither too much nor too little. Good professional listening may provide this sort of attachment experience.

In childhood, the secure base is used as a base for what Bowlby called 'a series of excursions', which continue throughout adulthood. As dependency decreases, the excursions become longer, so that eventually the dependent individual can exist without anxiety away from the attachment figure. Such excursions also provide safety for creative exploration and hypothesis-testing. In the same way as mental illness stimulates attachment behaviour, patients need a secure base from which to make a series of excursions back to a level of optimal function. The asylum function of a psychiatric institution is a good example of a secure base, which can provide a basis for cognitive and affective exploration, including the chance to make and learn from mistakes safely.

FEATURES OF ATTACHMENT-BASED PSYCHIATRIC CARE

Any attachment figure can modulate anxiety in a number of ways; by acting as an affective container, by providing information, and by providing consistent input. The affective containment aspect of attachment may be seen as similar to that maternal containment function described by Bion (1962). The primary care-giver helps the baby to develop a capacity to think and tolerate anxiety by using her own mental processes to hold and digest the baby's internal projections. In this way, the baby's first cognitive and affective fragments are understood and contained, thus reducing anxiety. This process also aids the baby in developing a capacity for abstract thought.

Impairment of thinking is a common feature of psychiatric illness, whether caused by psychotic or affective illness, or by anxiety disorders. It is plausible that, at an unconscious level, psychiatric staff fulfil a containing function for their patients. Care-givers may be internalised cognitively and affectively to produce a care-giver 'icon' (Kraemer, 1992), which can then be utilised by the patient to relieve anxiety.

Consciously, containment can be offered by empathic listening, which may be experienced as soothing. Providing information in a non-threatening way may also help to reduce anxiety. General information may be about the ward, the hospital or the course of any psychiatric illness. Specific information might be given about how mental illness affects a specific patient, or how the patient is experienced by others. Anxiety is reduced further by the development of trust, which itself is fostered by consistency of interaction. Consistency of staff input allows the patient some degree of predictability in a new anxiety-provoking situation. Listening, information-giving and consistency offer conscious cognitive containment of anxiety.

Insecure attachment patterns and patient responses

Attachments to mental health care professionals and institutions may persist long after an individual worker has left, or the institution closed down. Even when psychiatric care has been less than helpful, patients may continue to come for appointments and seek out help. Such attachment may reflect their neediness; however, it may also be a manifestation of the replication of insecure attachment patterns (Main and Goldwyn, 1989). Mental representations of attachment may affect the way individuals can make use of help that is offered. Dismissing individuals may find it difficult to engage with treatment. Preoccupied individuals may get stuck, find it difficult to move on, or act ambivalently towards offered care. Unresolved individuals may have difficulty in thinking about or managing the painful feelings aroused by treatment. By contrast, patients with a history of secure attachment in childhood are more likely to be compliant with medication, and to disclose more of their symptoms (Dozier, 1990).

It seems reasonable to conclude that many aspects of relationships between psychiatric patients and staff resemble attachment relationships. The patient, the mental health professionals and the institution all contribute to these relationships by an interactive process. This interactive process is seen in the clinical life of the unit; the problems that patients pose to staff, and the way staff respond, both consciously and unconsciously.

MANAGEMENT PROBLEMS AS ATTACHMENT BEHAVIOUR

Deliberate self-harm

If attachment bonds develop between psychiatric patients and staff, then problems might be expected at those times when attachment behaviour is stimulated, such as separations, or new threats to security. In general psychiatric units, the two most common situations are discharge, or loss of a specific worker – both examples of separations. Psychiatric patients may be fearful about leaving the ward to which they became attached when ill; worsening of symptoms is commonly seen before discharge, which may be seen as a form of protest. The most extreme forms of protest may be seen in those patients who deliberately harm themselves.

Miss A. was a 33-year-old woman with a long history of contact with psychiatric services. As a child, she had been raised by a mother with bipolar disorder, and an alcoholic father who was extremely physically abusive to all the children. She had spent much of her early life in different care settings. She was described by one psychiatrist as 'the angriest person I have ever seen'. Miss A. regularly sought extra unscheduled time with staff in the out-patient clinic, and refusal of her request would result in overdoses and self-harm.

Deliberate self-harming behaviours often occur following interaction with another person, usually one to whom the self-mutilator is attached and who may be threatening to leave. Such actions may be seen as pathological attachment behaviours, which are both an attempt to dissuade the care-giver from leaving, and a means of reducing arousal.

Disturbed behaviour may be a reaction to the loss of a specific attachment figure, such as a key nurse, even if feelings of attachment are not consciously recognised. Mental state deterioration has been observed in in-patients who have temporarily lost their consultant (Persaud and Meux, 1994).

Anger and violence

Distress and anxiety may also manifest as anger, which, together with anxiety, is a common manifestation of failed or insecure attachment (Bowlby, 1984). Anger may be expressed in order to dissuade the care-giver from leaving, as a protection of a relationship which is valuable to the angry person. A particular finding of interest is that anger may specifically be expressed towards care-givers (Main and George, 1985), suggesting that there is something about perceived failures of care-giving that may elicit anger.

Miss A. had made a therapeutic attachment to a member of the clinical team. They worked together, meeting regularly, for over two years. The team member wished to withdraw, and gave notice to Miss A. of her planned departure. Miss A. grabbed a pair of scissors, forcing the team member to shut the door and barricade it. Miss A. stood for some time outside the door, gouging out the wood with the scissors, and being verbally abusive. Eventually she had to be removed by security.

Understanding violence to health care professionals as attachment behaviour

Where mental health care professionals are seen as attachment figures, threats to relationships with them may produce anger and violence. Assaults on staff, or self-harming behaviour are associated with the diagnosis in individuals of some types of personality disorder. Personality disorder may be manifested as failure to make attachments, including engaging with psychiatric services. Attacks may be made on offered care, either indirectly by sabotaging treatment plans, or directly by assaults on staff. This can lead to rejection by staff and the termination of care. It is recognised that such patients are unpopular with mental health care professionals; as unpopular as they probably were with their original parents. Some of their maladaptive behaviours can be seen as traumatic re-enactments of earlier rejection and abuse (Van der Kolk, 1989).

Such behaviours may also represent an unconscious struggle for mastery of overwhelming affects, in the same way as attachment behaviour in infancy unconsciously reduces anxiety. Traumatic re-enactment functions as a projective measure, so that the victim remains a victim, and all their aggression is projected onto their aggressor. Identification with the aggressor offers another means of soothing and managing aggressive impulses. Projective identification, as a cognitive and affective strategy, is most likely to be used by those individuals who lacked an attachment figure who could contain and soothe their arousal. It is not surprising to find this primitive defence against anxiety in use on psychiatric wards. By this mechanism, care-givers may then be perceived as persecutory and aggressive. The reality of this perception for the patient should not be underestimated in terms of dangerousness; violence to staff may be understood by patients as an attempt to defend themselves against anxiety-inducing objects.

RESPENSES OF PROFESSIONALS: CLINICAL PRACTICE AND COUNTERTRANSFERENCE

Common psychiatric problems can be understood in attachment terms; there are many aspects of good professional practice in mental health which encourage attachment bonds to develop. In addition, professional carers themselves may have attachment histories which affect the relationships they form with patients. Attachment psychopathology in the staff may be just as problematic, and harder to detect.

It is known that many health care professionals have experience of illness in their own families. This may be a positive feature. However, negative family experiences of illness have been shown to be related to later occupational stress in health care professionals (Vaillant *et al.*, 1972; Firth Cozens, 1992).

Adults deprived of care in childhood may seek to provide it for others in their professional lives (Vaillant *et al.*, 1972). One manifestation of insecure attachment in children described by Bowlby is a style of relating called compulsive care-giving, whereby the child attends to the needs of others, and disregards their own. Bowlby suggested that children forced into this role develop a false adulthood, similar to the notion of false self proposed by Winnicott (1965).

It is possible that compulsive care-giving is a psychological style which may be found in a proportion of all health care professionals. This style may not be pathological *per se*; however, it is known that sick health care professionals are often reluctant to admit any difficulties, or seek help. Suppression of dependency needs leads to difficulties in acknowledging the demanding nature of the work. This can lead to denial of feelings generally, and specifically denial of the psychological needs of both patients and staff. Feelings of distress remain hidden and suppressed, leading to the use of pathological defences such as substance misuse to reduce anxiety, or to staff burn-out.

Maladaptive caring

Under stress, carers may develop maladaptive interpersonal strategies with patients; usually in the form of over-involvement with the patient's distress, or a tendency to dismiss it. Over-involved carers may need their patients to remain in a cared-for role, and find it difficult to allow patients to improve and regain independence. Over-involvement can result in boundary violations of various degrees; this is a common problem with those patients with abusive histories. Dismissal of distress can lead to rejection of patients, and intolerance of distress and dependence. The pejorative use of the term 'attention-seeking' also gives an idea of the wish to reject neediness experienced by some health care professionals.

Failure to address dependency needs can lead to anger (Bowlby, 1984), which fuels a wish to reject patients seen as 'troublesome'. Projections of anger and fear by patients are likely to resonate with the care-giver's own unconscious aggression. Care-givers may feel overwhelmed with feelings of fear and aggression, which are experienced as both alien and real. These strong countertransferential feelings may then be acted out, either overtly unprofessionally, or more commonly by covert use of professional structures, such as ward rounds or rigid enforcement of contracts (Main, 1977).

Mental health care professionals who have themselves survived frank abuse in childhood may act out more pathologically in the caring role. Such adults may become abusive themselves, identifying with the aggressor in the same way as was described for patients above. This may manifest itself as abuse of patients, either physical or sexual. Various public inquiries have shown that this can happen at either an individual or institutional level. A milder manifestation of such experiences may be inappropriate relationships with patients, transgressing professional boundaries. This is perhaps even more likely with patients who have been abused in childhood. Boundary violations and sexual exploitations of such patients by health care professionals is now recognised as a significant therapeutic problem (Gabbard, 1989).

THE INSTITUTION AS AN ATTACHMENT FIGURE

Mental health care institutions can be a positive attachment figure for patients, especially those who did not experience secure attachment in childhood. However, mental health care institutions may also fail to provide a secure base. Psychiatric institutions may be frightening in terms of architecture, atmosphere or ward population. The institutional environment may stimulate abnormal attachment behaviour, rather than reduce it. Attention-seeking behaviour may be related to a need for alleviation of anxiety and arousal, which is understandable from both an ethological perspective, and in terms of a patient's personal experience.

Institutional settings which infantilise and disempower patients will encourage regression and an expectation of 'special' care in the patients. If such expectations are both frustrated and criticised, then this increases confusion and anxiety in an already vulnerable patient. Ward regimes often encourage both dependence and independence simultaneously; so that an individual is 'ill' and in need of care, until they misbehave in some way and 'must take responsibility for themselves'.

Institutions may be ambivalent about the services they provide, encouraging staff to develop different types of treatment or support, then failing to provide structures to make them possible. This ambivalence presumably reflects that of the staff and the general public, especially in relation to difficult or violent patients. Lack of support for staff, both managerial and financial, may reduce institutional capacity to respond sensitively and appropriately to patients' needs. Inconsistency of staff, both in personal terms and in terms of staffing levels, also increases anxiety, while decreasing the capacity to contain it.

Other institutional factors operate at a wider level to stimulate abnormal attachment behaviour in patients. Therapeutic approaches which take a very particular kind of 'scientific' approach may be seen as defences against the emotional experience of being mentally ill (Main, 1977). An emphasis on pharmacological treatments of distress, when combined with a subtle (or not so subtle) denigration of empathic listening skills, means that staff are ill-equipped to modulate patient anxiety, or contain regressed behaviour. Involuntary detention may be experienced by patients as controlling and abusive, no matter how justified the detention on ethical and clinical grounds. This is particularly so for those patients who were 'detained' in care as children, after abuse by parents.

IMPLICATIONS FOR TREATMENT

Psychiatric care providers may not be able to alter radically the nature of patients' psychopathology. However, there are ways in which psychiatric environments, both physical and interpersonal, could be more containing of patient anxiety and arousal, and provide a safe base for patients to move to recovery and beyond.

The first step is to provide a secure base. This can be understood as the ward, the out-patient clinic or the buildings themselves. A secure base can offer affective containment and anxiety modulation by a multi-modal management strategy, which includes long-term psychological support, the appropriate use of the Mental Health Act, and appropriate medication. The aim of a clinical attachment-focused strategy would be to allow the patient to develop new skills in modulating their own anxiety, and examine maladaptive attachment patterns, in their own lives and on the ward. Such an approach also allows staff to understand disturbed behaviour as manifestations of severe anxiety and arousal in disabled individuals; and may also allow them to reflect on the aspects of their own attachments which contributed to their choice of a career in professional caring.

Attachment theory and research suggest that attachment behaviour can change in response to interpersonal experience (Fonagy et al., 1996). Work with non-human primates suggests that the behaviour of socially isolated monkeys may be improved after contact with 'therapist' monkeys. Vulnerable children may be protected by contact with one consistent parenting figure, and the presence of a confiding relationship is a protection against depression (Brown and Harris, 1978). Personality disorders may be responsive to treatment approaches that take account of attachment needs, behaviours and bonds (Linehan, 1992).

Understanding disturbed ward behaviour in the light of attachment theory may help in the management of such behaviour. A proactive emphasis on anxiety and arousal reduction, combined with careful planning of separations and losses on wards, might help to reduce tension and violence; at least as much as the provision of courses for staff in control and restraint.

Secure attachment fostering change

Miss A. was offered fixed appointments with the team psychiatrist, and open, but limited 'drop-in' time with a nurse who knew her well. Close adherence to boundaries, combined with a flexible capacity to respond at times of distress, and appropriate use of medication, helped contain Miss A.'s distress, and lead to a reduction in violence to others, and to herself. When the team psychiatrist left the team after three years, Miss A. was warned well in advance. At their last meeting, she was able to thank him for the help she had received, and express grief that he was going.

The positive effects of a professional carer 'being with', rather than 'doing to' patients is well known. This is likely to be particularly true for those with histories of failed attachment. Confiding in someone, telling one's story and being listened to are potent modulators of anxiety. The traumatic stress litera- ture has shown the value of narrative in reducing fear in all forms of psycho- therapy, cognitive and dynamic. Cultural identities are built and sustained in tales, stories and myths. It can be therapeutic just to listen to stories of depriva-tion and distress; there is a danger that current psychiatric practice offers little or no space for recounting painful experiences. Attachment theory suggests that long-term listening may be important for those patients who have distress-ing stories to tell.

CONCLUSION

Attachment theory continues to develop, both empirically and clinically. It has demonstrated its value; first, as a theory which combines ethology, neurobiology and individual psychology; and second, as a means of examining empirically hypotheses based on psychodynamic clinical work. Psychodynamic approaches to general psychiatric practice, based on attach-ment theory, allow for the recognition of both the patient's and the profes-sional's subjectivity, and an understanding of the importance of that subjectiv-ity for therapeutic relationships. Violence and other negative staff–patient interactions need to be understood in the light of patient's previous attach-ments, and replication of those attachments with staff. Attachment theory offers possibilities for research into understanding staff–patient relationships in general psychiatric hospitals. It also offers a way of thinking about change.

REFERENCES

Ainsworth, M., Blehar, M.C., Waters, E., *et al.* (1978). *Patterns of Attachment: A Psychobiological Study of the Strange Situation.* Hillsdale, NJ: Erlbaum.

Bion, W. (1962). *Learning from Experience.* London: Heinemann.

Bowlby, J. (1979). On knowing what you are not supposed to know and feeling what you are not supposed to feel. *Canadian Journal of Psychiatry,* 24, p.403–408.

Bowlby, J.(1984). Violence in the family as a disorder of the attachment and care-giving systems. *American Journal of Psychoanalysis,* 44, p.9–27.

Bowlby, J. (1988). *A Secure Base: Clinical Applications of Attachment Theory.* London: Routledge.

Bremner, J.D., Southwick, S., Johnson, O., *et al.* (1993). Child physical abuse and combat related PTSD in Vietnam veterans. *American Journal of Psychiatry,* 150, p.235–239.

Brown, G. and Harris, T. (1978). *The Social Origins of Depression.* London: Tavistock.

Dozier, M. (1990). Attachment organisation and treatment use for adults with serious psychopathological disorders. *Development and Psychopathology,* 2, p.47–60.

Firth Cozens, J. (1992). The role of early family experiences in the perception of organisational stress: fusing clinical and organisational perspectives. *Journal of Occupational and Organisational Psychology,* 65, p.61–75.

Fonagy, P., Steele, M., Steele, H., *et al.* (1996). The relationship of attachment status, psychiatric classification and response to psychotherapy. *Journal of Consulting and Clinical Psychology,* 64, p.22–31.

Gabbard, G. (1989). *Sexual Exploitation in Professional Relationships.* Washington, DC: American Psychiatric Press.

Garland, C. (1991). External disasters and the internal world: an approach to psychotherapeutic understanding of survivors. In J. Holmes, ed., *Textbook of Psychotherapy in Psychiatric Practice.* London: Churchill Livingstone. p.507–532.

Kraemer, G. (1992). A psychobiological theory of attachment. *Behavioural and Brain Sciences*, 15, p.493–511.

Linehan, M., Armstrong, H.E., Suarez, A., *et al.* (1992). Cognitive-behavioural treatment of chronically parasuicidal borderline patients. *Archives of General Psychiatry*, 48, p.1060–1064.

Main, M. and George, C. (1985). Responses of abused and disadvantaged toddlers to distress in age-mates: a study in a day care setting. *Developmental Psychology*, 21, p.407–412.

Main, M., Kaplan, N. and Cassidy, J. (1985). Security in infancy, childhood and adulthood: a move to the level of representation. *Monographs of the Society for Research into Child Development*, 50, p.66–104.

Main, M. and Goldwyn, R. (1989). *Adult Attachment Rating and Classification System.* Department of Psychology. University of California, Berkeley, CA.

Main, T. (1977). Traditional psychiatric defences against close encounters with patients. *Canadian Psychiatric Association Journal*, 22, p.457–466.

Mullen, P.E., Martin, L., Anderson, C., *et al.* (1993). Child sexual abuse and mental health in adult life. *British Journal of Psychiatry*, 163, p.721–730.

Ogata, S., Silk, K., Goodrich, S., *et al.* (1990). Childhood sexual abuse and physical abuse in adult patients with borderline personality disorder. *American Journal of Psychiatry*, 147, p.1008–1013.

Parker, G. (1983). Parental 'affectionless control' as an antecedent to adult depression. *Archives of General Psychiatry*, 40, p.956–960.

Parkes, C.M. (1991). 'Attachment, bonding and psychiatric problems after bereavement in adult life'. In C.M. Parkes, J. Stevenson-Hinde and P. Harris, (eds), *Attachment Across the Life Cycle.* London: Routledge. p.268–292.

Patrick, M., Hobson, P., Castle, D., *et al.* (1994). Personality disorder and the mental representation of early social experience. *Development and Psychopathology*, 6, p.375–388.

Persaud, R.D. and Meux. C.J. (1994). The psychopathology of authority and its loss: the effect on a ward of losing a consultant psychiatrist. *British Journal of Medical Psychology*, 67, p.1–11.

Rutter, M. (ed.) (1988). 'Attachment and the development of social relationships.' In *Scientific Foundations of Developmental Psychiatry.* Washington, DC: American Psychiatric Press. p.267–279.

Rutter, M. (1995). Clinical implications of attachment theory: retrospect and prospect. *Journal of Child Psychology and Psychiatry*, 36, p.549–571.

Vaillant, G., Sobowale, N. and McArthur, B. (1972). Some psychological vulnerabilities in physicians. *New England Journal of Medicine*, 287, p.372–375.

Van der Kolk, B. (1989). The compulsion to repeat the trauma: re-enactment, revictimisation and masochism. *Psychiatric Clinics of North America*, 12, p.389–411.

Van der Kolk, B., Perry, C. and Herman, J. (1991). Childhood origins of self-destructive behaviour. *American Journal of Psychiatry*, 148, p.1665–1671.

Van Ijzendoorn, M.H. and Bakermans Kranenburg, M. (1996). Attachment representations in mothers, fathers, adolescents and clinical groups: A meta-analytic search for normative data. *Journal of Consulting and Clinical Psychology*, 64, p.8–21.

Weiss, R. (1991). 'The attachment bond in childhood and adulthood.' In C.M. Parkes, J. Stevenson-Hinde and P. Harris, (eds), *Attachment Across the Life Cycle*. London: Routledge. p.66–76.

Winnicott, D. (1965). 'Ego distortion in terms of true and false self.' In D. Winnicott, (ed.), *The Maturational Process and the Facilitating Environment*. London: Hogarth. p.140–152.

10

In the Prison of
Severe Personality Disorder[*]

Kingsley Norton
1997

· ·

Editors' reflections

The author of this paper is one of our national experts in working with personality disorder, especially in groups and residential settings. Like Scott Henderson, he assumes that there is meaning in the individual's anti-social or unpopular behaviours and suggests that staff need help to understand this. If the staff can understand what is being re-enacted with them, and resist acting like punitive or seductive carers, then they can help service users with severe personality disorders 'break out' of their prison.

· ·

> Treatment of the patient, who suffers from a disturbance of social relationships, cannot be…regarded as satisfactory unless it is undertaken within a framework of *social reality* which can provide him with opportunities for attaining fuller social insight and for expressing and modifying his emotional drives according to the demands of *real life*…full opportunity must be available for identifying and analysing the interpersonal barriers which stand in the way of participation in a full community life. (Main, 1946: p.67; emphases added)

[*]   Originally published in *Journal of Forensic Psychiatry and Psychology*, 8, 2, 285–298. Reprinted here by permission of Taylor and Francis.

Abstract

Interpersonal barriers frequently stand in the way of the successful treatment of patients suffering from severe personality disorder (SPD). Often this stems from a failure to distinguish accurately between the patient's surface behavioural manifestations and his or her inner mental states. Misinterpreting the SPD patient's gross behaviour may thus result in unsuccessful clinical encounters because of the absence of empathic contact with the patient and a resultant insubstantial therapeutic alliance. Inpatient staff's failure to see through and beyond their SPD patients' behavioural facades means that such patients continue to feel marginalised and misunderstood, and that staff become no wiser in understanding their patients as individuals.

The SPD patient's strong negative emotion and its interpersonal behavioural concomitants may be erroneously equated with no progress, deterioration, or even 'badness' and his or her compliant behaviour may be mistaken for therapeutic progress and psychological change. Clinical decisions regarding the discharge or transfer of SPD patients, based on such grounds, are likely to be unsafe. If staff recognise SPD patients' profound problems in identifying and communicating their painful mental states, they are better able to help them to give up the self-defeating and anti-social coping strategies and defences that are erected by patients in order to deal with such states. Via the removal of such barriers, some SPD patients may be freed from a metaphorical 'prison', which is only part of their own making.

Clinical material from some of Henderson Hospital's SPD inpatients is presented to exemplify the behavioural camouflage assumed by such patients thereby masking their inner states and the consequent interpersonal difficulties encountered in their treatment. Aspects of the therapeutic community (TC) method of identifying and analysing the difficulties, in particular the availability and use of the 'social reality' of the setting, are discussed. Implications for other non-TC, inpatient settings are considered so that the 'social reality' found therein can be put to greater therapeutic use.

BACKGROUND

The overt behaviour of many patients suffering from severe personality disorder (SPD) does not permit an accurate evaluation of the psychological inmate (Kernberg, 1984). It acts as a barrier which blocks the possibility of an authentic emotional relationship. Although the outward appearance may vary – for example it may be intimidating, seductive, buoyant, or reserved – each behavioural style of relating serves to regulate the emotional distance between the SPD patient and others, so that the other person is maintained on the 'outside'.

Thus it is that the SPD patient's observable behaviour not only masks what the psychological inmate is thinking or feeling but fails to convey that inmate's ambivalence about, and difficulty with, verbalising the true nature of his or her internal predicament.

INTERPERSONAL BARRIERS

One of the goals of the inpatient therapeutic community (TC) is to identify the SPD patient's interpersonal barriers to participation in a full community life (Main, 1946).

The TC works to achieve this aim through the safe transformation of the patient's 'intrapsychic impairment into interpersonal discord' (Tucker *et al.*, 1987). This therapeutic approach is required since many SPD patients are not able to verbalise their problems. Thus, they need to present 'of' themselves rather than 'from within' (Brooke, 1994).

Recognising the SPD patient's difficulty with verbalising needs for help, the TC provides an elaborate treatment programme (see Table 1). This offers opportunities for the interpersonal enactment of the internal difficulty and also for its detection (Norton, 1997). Monitoring for evidence of interpersonal enactment requires paying close attention to the whole 24-hour period, including both formal therapy sessions and the unstructured (sociotherapy) time (Norton, 1995). Once detected, the causes and consequences of interpersonal enactments can be explored and analysed in relation to the SPD patient's underlying intrapsychic conflict (Main, 1983).

The democratic TC method of identifying and analysing the SPD patient's interpersonal difficulties relies on the active participation of the patient's peers as well as of staff. It requires a much greater collaboration between these two 'systems' of the inpatient environment than is usually found in general or secure psychiatric settings – 'communalism' (Rapoport, 1960). Such a collaborative endeavour is sustained by the relative prominence of group-based treatments over individual psychotherapy. It is achieved also by the joint participation of patients and staff in non-therapy aspects, which are usually the preserve of hospital staff, such as the ordering and cooking of the patients' food; and responsibility for minor maintenance of the fabric of the building and upkeep of the hospital's garden (Jones, 1952).

The patients' acceptance of responsibility for a range of practical (as well as some emotional) tasks central to the smooth daily running of the unit potentially provides staff with evidence of how patients are likely to interact in real-life situations, on the 'outside'. Whether and how such responsibility is accepted thus provides material for discussion and exploration within the formal psychotherapy sessions (Mahony, 1979). Insights gained there may suggest changes in the SPD patient's attitudes or behaviour which can be experimented with during the unstructured time (Whiteley, 1979). In this way, the unit's formal psychotherapy sessions and unstructured sociotherapy can complement one another (Edelson, 1970). To maximise the complementarity of psychotherapy and sociotherapy, however, requires effective communication between the patients and staff as well as between staff themselves. This necessitates a flattening of the traditional staff–patient hierarchy (Jones, 1952) and relies on a culture that is confrontative and supportive (Norton, 1992a) rather than simply condemning or condoning, through a collusive silence and the keeping of secrets (Norton and Dolan, 1995).

Monitoring, both the attendance at formal therapy sessions and also the undertaking of domestic tasks involved in running the unit, during the unstructured time, is carried out by patients themselves, as part of a range of 'real tasks' (see below). Absences or other irregularities, including excessive zeal, are communicated in the daily 'community meeting' of the whole TC, as part of an ongoing 'reality confrontation' (Rapport, 1960; Norton, 1996). In this way, individual SPD patients are challenged with evidence of their personal issues that block meaningful interpersonal contact with others. Such a challenge is carried out in an atmosphere of enquiry, with the emphasis laid on understanding rather than on punishment (Main, 1983; Norton, 1992a).

Even such a conducive therapeutic atmosphere does not permit some SPD patients to feel safe enough emotionally to enact their problems interpersonally, let alone to be sufficiently composed to verbalise them. These patients are especially difficult to treat because their 'prison wall' behaviour is particularly opaque and impenetrable. Neither staff nor other patients know what is happening to the psychological inmate behind the 'prison walls'. With them there is little or no detectable evidence of their psychopathology either within formal therapy sessions or during the unstructured time (Norton, 1997). Such patients are often engaged only in an 'illusory alliance' (Meloy, 1988) which has seriously limited predictive value for staff in helping the latter to decide how these patients might fare in another environment, outside of hospital.

	Monday	Tuesday	Wednesday	Thursday	Friday	Saturday	Sunday
9.15 – 10.30	'9.15' Community meeting						
10.30 – 11.00	**Morning break**						
11.00 – 12.00	Small group psychotherapy	Reviews and cleaning; elections or community projects	Small group psychotherapy or leavers' group	Welfare group, probation group, or visitors' group	Small group psychotherapy		
12.00 – 13.30	**Lunch break**						
13.30 – 14.00 14.15 or 14.30 – 16.30	Surgery Psychodrama or art therapy	Cleaning Selection, community work group or housing group	Art therapy or psychodrama	Gardening and maintenance, art work group, or welfare group			
16.45 – 17.00	**Afternoon break**						
17.00 – 17.15		'Handover' to night staff (Two residents and two day staff)					
18.00 – 19.00		Women's group		Men's group			
19.00 – 21.00	**Community meal**						
21.15 – 22.05	'Tens' group (optional)						
22.15 – 23.00	Summit meeting (Top three residents and staff)						
23.00	Night round (Top three residents and staff)						

Table 1 – Treatment programme in the therapeutic community

CASE EXAMPLES

Anne – bland or jolly

Anne suffers from SPD. She self-mutilates. Early during her inpatient therapeutic community (TC) stay, her self-harming behaviour baffled both the staff and her peers because it appeared to arise out of the blue. There was no direct evidence of upset or disturbance presented during formal psychotherapy sessions and no indirect evidence from any obvious interpersonal discord occurring at other times. Neither patients nor staff knew anything of an internal motivating state for her self-injurious behaviour. No empathic contact with Anne was possible.

After 3 months or so in the TC, Anne was able to report that she self-mutilated either when feeling, in her own words, 'frighteningly calm' or else when 'wound up with a whirlwind of thoughts' going around in her head. Cutting or burning herself, she claimed, afforded her relief from both these states of mind. Anne's inner mental frenzy or, alternatively, her unnatural calm, however, continued to lie behind a bland exterior or a false gaiety – different forms of 'prison walls'. The distancing effect on others of both facades only served to reinforce Anne's sense of alienation from them and her dependence on self-harming behaviour for intermittent relief from her mental pain.

After 8 months of her inpatient stay, Anne still finds verbalising something of her internal mental states to be an alien experience. She feels vulnerable, believing that others will exploit her for speaking her mind, since she construes this as a sign of 'weakness'. In fact, the effect of Anne's verbalising her distress has allowed others to offer emotional support to her and also to confront her when she self-harms, instead of her asking them for support. She is learning that other people do not necessarily take advantage of her when she reveals her emotional distress or the inner disturbance she is experiencing. Beginning to trust others, Anne feels she has gained a greater sense of personal mastery and more freedom to choose how to behave, both in relation to herself and to others. This includes a greater emotional transparency, which allows others more access to her inner world. She has begun to talk about her disrupted childhood during which she attended more than twenty schools, as the family followed in the wake of her father's peripatetic lifestyle, trailing after him around the country.

Bob – aggressive and angry

Bob, another SPD inpatient, has served several prison sentences for serious violent and sexual offences. His criminal career began early when his prostitute mother schooled him in stealing from her clients. A compulsion to seek fights was his presenting problem. This was often enacted in nightclubs, which Bob visited with the intention of provoking the toughest-looking male in the place. Bob was usually successful in this venture, although by no means always did he come off the worst in the ensuing fight, despite this being his stated intention.

In the TC setting, it gradually became clear that Bob managed his psychic pain by setting up interpersonal confrontations that were at risk of dangerous escalation. The inpatient TC environment provided him with plenty of opportunities to do so, both within and between formal psychotherapy sessions. It was therefore important that early evidence of confrontation was detected and explored, before escalation became established.

Exploration of such evidence has revealed that it is when Bob is particularly fearful and vulnerable that he feels impelled to provoke a fight. As a result of this insight, others are starting to be able to resist rising to Bob's provocative bait. Bob himself is starting to feel worse. He is also relieved, however, that others are beginning to see beyond his intimidating 'prison wall' behaviour to the vulnerable inmate inside. Such relief was previously available to him only through the physical exhaustion of fighting and being physically injured.

Carol – quiet and charming

Carol suffers from SPD. In spite of some obvious difference, she shares important features of behavioural camouflage with Bob and Anne. Unlike Bob, she is quiet and self-effacing in most of her interpersonal dealings, playing little obvious part in the hospital's TC life. Like Anne, she reveals precious little of a personal kind either in formal psychotherapy or in the unstructured time she spends in the hospital. She uses her charm to deflect any probing enquiry about herself.

Inside, Carol is frequently 'wound up', just like Anne. One of her escapes from this state of mind is to seek violent sexual contact, as a victim, while away from the hospital. Afterwards she feels exhausted, humiliated, dirty and ashamed. However, this provides her with a sense of relief, as did Bob's fights for him. It appears to be this, which reinforces the particular form of Carol's behaviour, which began in her early teens when she ran away from home to escape a violent and sexually abusive relationship with her stepfather.

The next stage for Carol is to identify what makes her feel 'wound up'. This will require a deeper level of interaction with others in the TC. Already Carol is beginning to understand that her reports of sexual victimisation are upsetting and even offensive to some of the other patients. She thus knows that her actions have an effect on others, not just on herself. She is consequently under pressure from her peers to speak when she feels 'wound up', in order to try to understand more about the origins and nature of this internal state, and not to take herself away from the hospital.

Danny – cool and mechanical

Danny's hands, arms and neck are heavily scarred. Of his siblings, he had borne the brunt of his alcoholic father's violence. Danny suffers from severe SPD characterised, amongst other attributes, by self-mutilation, violence to others and serious misuse of illicit drugs and alcohol. He complains of being 'treated like a robot', in the past by his family and currently by fellow residents for whom he caters excessively and behind whom he cleans up. He voices his complaint, however, without appropriate emphasis and his words do not translate into actions. For example, he appears unable to restrain his impulse to offer his services when volunteers for cooking the community's evening meal (for more than 25 people) are asked for. This is in spite of his 'complaints' that he is taken for granted. Following occasional evenings out of the TC, Danny regales his peers with fantastic tales of frightening and heroic happenings. Nobody seems interested in listening to him.

Danny appears to participate actively in the TC but he remains essentially emotionally dislocated with no meaningful relationship to other patients or staff. Nobody takes Danny's concerns or 'tales' seriously. Unlike Anne's, his self-harming stopped completely after admission. Unlike Bob, he has avoided authentic confrontation with others in the TC. There is no interpersonal enactment, either aggressive or sexual, which can be detected either during formal therapy or the unstructured time. It is as if he has no intra-psychic conflict or interpersonal difficulties, even though his forensic history and physical scars clearly tell a different story. Initially, staff mistakenly concluded that Danny's apparent conscientiousness represented an authentic therapeutic alliance. Like many other SPD patients, the above patients have features of their inner mental states, as well as some aspects of their contradictory, or masking, 'prison walls', appearance and behaviour in common. A number of them, like Anne, spontaneously use the metaphor of the 'whirlwind' to refer to their internal states. It is as if, for much of the time, such patients are caught up in a whirlwind at the interface of the winds and the eye of the storm. Thus there can be spiralling gales of out-of-control thoughts (sometimes associated with 'highs' of mood), at one moment and the unnatural calm of the eye (in which they feel paralysed, empty, or forever falling), in the next. Neither state feels comfortable. In being mentally buffeted by the swirling winds, patients crave the eye's calm. Once out of the wind, however, the despairing emptiness of the cavernous eye is experienced as intolerable. There is a craving for escape to relieve the unbearable strain of nothingness.

In one domain of the whirlwind there is difficulty with thinking – thoughts are racing. Thus the SPD patient is unable to concentrate because of an inability to apprehend and focus on one thought or feeling. In the other domain there is a mental paralysis in the moment (see Sims, 1988, for abnormalities of experience of the passage of time), with no energy to anticipate the next moment – down in the doldrums (Lambert, 1981). By their own account, much of the maladaptive behaviour of these patients stems from abortive attempts to escape from the control of these countervailing emotional weather systems. However, the result of the behaviour is often only a temporary shift from one extreme to the other. It is experienced as worthwhile, however, since it serves to reinforce what often has become an addictive system (see Joseph, 1982).

With other SPD patients, such as Danny, their habitual time-space may be away from the area where the wall of winds meets the eye and, instead, in the eye of the whirlwind itself. So, Esther Greenwood, Sylvia Plath's fictitious heroine of *The Bell Jar*, describes herself near the start of the novel:

> I just bumped from my hotel to work and to parties and from parties to my hotel and back to work like a number trolley-bus. I guess I should have been excited the way most girls were, but I couldn't get myself to react. I felt very still and very empty, *the way the eye of a tornado must feel*, moving dully along in the middle of the surrounding hullabaloo.

> (Plath, 1963; emphasis added)

The situation with Danny, not to mention that of Esther Greenwood (or of Sylvia Plath?), reveals how alienated from the world such people often feel, akin to the experiencing chronic feelings of de-personalisation. Much of the time, SPD patients feel as if imprisoned in a 'frighteningly calm' or deadening inner psychic world. They are cut off from the outer world and devoid of full contact with others. When available, physical and chemical solutions to their problematic inner states (for example, via self-mutilation or drugs misuse) may be utilised to excite or energise. These shocking methods are used since ordinary (non-abusive) human interaction often fails to relieve the pain of the inner state. Everyday inpatient ward routines and traditional psychiatric interpersonal activity may thus not make any impact on such SPD patients as they move dully along in the middle of the surrounding (psychiatric) hullabaloo!

After several months in the TC, Danny was beginning to change. He confided in another patient that he had taken a serious overdose the previous day. This not only had endangered his life but it represented the breaking of one of the TC's major rules, proscribing damage to self. The other patient informed the senior patients whose task it was to call an emergency meeting in order to enquire after and explore this untoward event.

During the meeting, Danny was confronted with this information. Grudgingly he admitted to its truth and, following this confession, other patients revealed that Danny had also confided in them. It transpired, however, that he had provided each of them with a significantly different account of events. These patients were all outraged both by the inconsistency of Danny's accounts and also by the fact that they had each believed every detail. As if to add insult to injury, Danny then mentioned that he had also self-mutilated, subsequent to feeling guilty about the secrets he was keeping from the majority of the community's members.

It was pointed out to Danny that his self-pitying tone, in relaying this new information, was misplaced. His peers were able to say, with considerable feeling, how annoyed and betrayed they were left feeling. They had felt devalued by Danny's recourse to behavioural means of communicating distress and obtaining relief.

Danny appeared shocked by the strength of the community's reaction. Later this had the effect of making him question his view of himself as a habitual victim. When all of this was processed in the formal psychotherapy sessions, he began to realise that not only did others' behaviour affect him emotionally but that his affected them similarly. He saw that his secretiveness and his mistrustful attitude, of which he was previously largely unaware, was part of a repeating pattern of relating in his family and within other of his intimate relationships. Danny now realised that he had contributed to the failure of some relationships in the past. This made him start to question his mechanistic view of himself and others and the roots of such attitudes in his earlier experiences of being actually victimised.

MAXIMISING 'SOCIAL REALITY' IN NON-TC SETTING

Real interactions

For inpatients such as Danny, the democratic TC's response to their 'acting out' means not being confronted solely by a response from staff, which may be affected or artifical, since they are constrained by the demands of their professional role (Norton and Dolan, 1995), but rather being on the receiving end of powerful emotional feedback from their peers and involved in 'real interactions'. Patients are left in no doubt about the impact of their behaviour on others, whether it is negative or positive. The communicating of positive feedback also carries more weight if it derives from the patient's peer group who can freely give vent to positive feelings towards a fellow community member. Staff are also constrained by their professional codes in terms of how and how far they convey warmth and congratulations to patients.

The reality of the interactions on offer, in such a TC setting, is a reflection of the emotional directness of the interpersonal expression. This directness comes especially from the patient's peer group and it is facilitated by the prominence of group-based treatment ingredients (Norton, 1996). However, it derives also from the speed of the TC's response to the patient, which guarantees that the emotional response is fresh. This is importantly provided by strategically placed 'after-groups' and by the facility of an 'emergency meeting' which can be convened at any time, whether by day or night (Norton, 1996).

In theory, it is possible to maximise these two aspects, directness and speediness of response, in any inpatient treatment setting, although not necessarily to the same degree in each. Thus, the use of group treatments can facilitate the peer group of patients to 'speak their minds' by increasing their self-confidence in addressing both staff members and also other patients seen by them as higher in the social hierarchy of the ward.

Real tasks

More decision-making can be delegated to ward patients and the members of the multi-disciplinary team who are on duty at a particular time. This can result in more power being invested in such personnel who are therefore better able to deal with not only any emergency situation but also more mundane matters, particularly outside normal working hours.

In many inpatient environments, it would be feasible to consider an evolutionary change towards such empowerment provided it were made clear how far and for what purpose the authority was delegated to the staff sub-team and to the patients (Norton, 1992a). With such a change, the 'social reality' of the ward comprising staff and patients (Main, 1946), would be increased with potential therapeutic benefit. A single example of the effect of an apparently trivial change in the distribution of authority and power may illustrate the point.

In a secure ward environment, run according to traditional (non-TC) lines, a weekly ward group meeting of all inpatients and ward staff was started. This was at the instigation of the nurse manager in overall charge of this and other secure wards. She had felt inundated with demands on her time by ward staff asking her to attend to a range of practical matters and complaints. In particular, there seemed to be a chronic shortage of electric light-bulbs on this particular ward. The manager believed that her life would be made easier if the patients' grumbles, and hence those of the ward staff, could be contained by the weekly meeting.

There were other shortages on this ward, however, and other complaints, albeit largely unspoken. Thus the regular ward staff felt under stress due to chronic staff shortages, which necessitated the employment of a succession of temporary staff to fill the vacant posts. The result was that the permanent staff were always needed to take charge of the ward and it fell to temporary staff to fulfil most of the other functions, including that of escorting patients who were granted permission to leave the ward. The temporary staff themselves had complaints. These centred on the fact that, although on duty during escort activities, they were expected to pay any expenses incurred, such as paying for their own cups of coffee or bus fares.

At the ward's third weekly meeting, one of the quieter female patients asked why the temporary ward staff could not buy a supply of light-bulbs. The permanent staff indicated there was no budget for this purpose. The patient persisted, however, by asking them why this was so. Initially inflamed by this question, the staff resolved in their own after-group meeting, during which they reviewed the earlier ward meeting, to ask the same question of the ward manager. Having done so, they were surprised to receive the necessary authorisation from her to manage the relevant budget themselves. This information was communicated back to the patients in the following ward meeting.

At that meeting, another patient suggested that he would be able to shop for the light-bulbs, when next 'on parole'. This offer was discussed at the ward round where it was agreed that such a task-centred activity, with appropriate escort, would be in the interests of the patient's rehabilitation, as well as of use to the ward itself. The escorting staff were glad to hear of the change of policy because it meant that they were no longer having to 'kill time' with patients, sitting in local coffee bars trying to make polite conversation. Instead, the staff were asked to observe the patient and to report on the real-life interactions – how the patients interacted with the shopkeeper, handled money; behaved generally in terms of appropriate social behaviour.

Staff and patients on the ward felt empowered, as a result of the small change in the direction of normal 'social reality'. They valued their direct involvement in the pursuit of 'real tasks', part of ordinary social life and part of the 'real life' of the ward itself. At least some of the frustration in the ward system and within the relationship between the ward staff and their manager lessened. In the light of the changes in policy, staff felt more aware of some of their patients' actual psychosocial capabilities.

CONCLUSION

The everyday 'social reality' of the inpatient setting is often ignored and seldom conceived of as an influential factor which may promote or hinder therapy. The democratic TC method aims to maximise the therapeutic potential of the hospital's total human environment by harnessing this to the structured programme of formal psychotherapy taking place therein. This requires an organisational structure that maximises effective communication and collaboration between staff and patients, as well as between staff. To achieve this, staff and patients need to be empowered so they can play as full a part in the 'social reality' as is appropriate to the particular unit. One important result is that more SPD patients can be engaged in an authentic therapeutic alliance.

Creating the potential for empathic contact with SPD patients and for their more genuine engagement in treatment is not only difficult to achieve, especially in secure settings, but often not welcomed by the patients themselves. They are ambivalent about release from a solitary confinement which has also provided them, in the past, with a degree of reliable solace from an inner 'whirlwind' reality. Staff therefore need to know the various, sometimes subtle, ways in which their patient's incarceration can be deliberately or inadvertently continued, including via staff's own attitudes and unwitting actions.

To facilitate the safe release of SPD patients from this form of internal imprisonment, non-TC inpatient therapeutic environments need to establish within themselves more of outside life's ordinary social reality and organisational complexity. This is easier said than done. It requires an overarching treatment philosophy or model, which integrates the therapeutic aims of the formal therapy ingredients with those of the unstructured time. It also requires that some of the tasks (both therapeutic and non-therapeutic) traditionally carried out by staff are delegated to patients.

The above organisational structures, when appropriately monitored, can afford staff better opportunities to observe their patients within interactions of the kind the patients are likely to encounter post-discharge. As a result, staff are in a position to make more accurate predictions for the later resettlement of their patients into the wider community (or at a lower level of inpatient security). Thus, the compliant behaviour of some SPD patients will be less often mistaken for clinical improvement or personality maturation and some of the expressions of verbal, as opposed to physical, aggression by SPD patients may be identified as aspects of healthy change and development.

ACKNOWLEDGEMENT

This paper is based upon one delivered by the author at a conference entitled 'Inpatient treatment of personality disordered patients' at the Cassel Hospital, Richmond, Surrey on 30 June 1995.

REFERENCES

Brooke, R. (1994). Assessment for Psychotherapy: Clinical Interactions of Self Cohesion and Self Pathology. *British Journal of Psychotherapy*, 10(3), 317–30.

Edelson, M. (1970). *Sociotherapy and Psychotherapy*. Chicago: University of Chicago Press.

Jones, M. (1952). *Social Psychiatry*. London: Tavistock Publications.

Joseph, B. (1982). Addiction to Near Death. *International Journal of Psychoanalysis*, 63, 449–56.

Kernberg, O.F. (1984). *Severe Personality Disorders: Psychotherapeutic Strategies*. London: Yale University Press.

Lambert, K. (1981). *Analysis, Repair and Individuation*. London: Academic Press.

Mahony, N. (1979). 'My Stay and Change at the Henderson Therapeutic Community.' In R.D. Hinshelwood and N. Manning, eds. *Therapeutic Communities: Reflections and Progress*. London: Routledge & Kegan Paul.

Main, T. (1946). The Hospital as a Therapeutic Institution. *Bulletin of the Meninger Clinic*, 10, 66–8.

Main, T. (1983). 'The Concept of the Therapeutic Community: Variations and Vicissitudes'. In M. Pines, ed. *The Evolution of Group Analysis*. London: Routledge & Kegan Paul.

Meloy, J.R. (1988). *The Psychopathic Mind: Origins, Dynamics and Treatment*. New Jersey: Jason Aronson Inc.

Norton, K.R.W. (1992a). A Culture of Enquiry: its Preservation or Loss. *Therapeutic Communities*, 13(1), 3–26.

Norton, K.R.W. (1992b). Personality Disordered Individuals: The Henderson Hospital model of treatment. *Criminal Behaviour and Mental Health*, 2, 180–91.

Norton, K.R.W. (1995). 'Personality Disordered Forensic Patients and the Therapeutic Community.' In C. Cordess and M. Cox, eds. *Forensic Psychotherapy*. London: Jessica Kingsley Publishers.

Norton, K.R.W. (1996). 'How Therapeutic Communities Work.' In G. Edwards and C. Dare, eds. *Psychotherapy, Psychological Treatments and the Addictions*. Cambridge: Cambridge University Press.

Norton, K.R.W. (1997). In-patient Psychotherapy: Integrating the Other 23 Hours. *Current Medical Literature – Psychiatry* 8(2), pp.31–37.

Norton, K.R.W. and Dolan, B.M. (1995). Acting Out and the Institutional Response. *Journal of Forensic Psychiatry*, 6(2), 317–32.

Plath, S. (1963). *The Bell Jar*. London: Heinemann.

Rapport, R. (1960). *The Community as Doctor*. London: Tavistock.

Sims, A. (1988). *Symptoms in the Mind: an Introduction to Descriptive Psychopathology*. London: Ballière Tindall.

Tucker, L., Banner, S.F., Wagner, S., Harlan, D. and Sher, I. (1987). Long-term Hospital Treatment of Borderline Patients: a Descriptive Outcome Study. *American Journal of Psychiatry*, 153(12), 1593–7.

Whitely, J.S. (1979). *Group Approaches in Psychiatry*. London: Routledge and Kegan Paul, pp.115–16.

Points for reflective practice

- What does 'borderline' mean to you?

- Can you recall times during your work with service users when hateful feelings have been aroused in you? And when you have felt afraid?

- What is it about these contacts with service users, or the service users themselves, which have generated these feelings?

- What do you 'do' with these feelings?

- Are there service users in your care who are (or have been) 'malignantly alienated'? What factors are present in the service user, the staff and the organisation that have contributed to this process?

- How do you feel when service users in your care act violently, towards themselves or towards others? What is your response to them? How do other staff members react? And the organisation respond? How could this be done differently?

- Are there service users in your care that you feel you have a 'special' or different relationship with, as opposed to other service users or staff? What is it about these service users that has evoked this feeling in you?

- Can you identify any current or past splits between staff over the treatment or management of a service user? What is being re-enacted here? What is it about the service user that may be influencing staff reactions?

Part III

Treatment and Management

11

Murmurs of Discontent: Treatment and Treatability of Personality Disorder[*]

Gwen Adshead
2001

Editors' reflections

We have all met patients who are described as 'untreatable', which allows professionals then to refuse patients services. Yet this is not an approach we take to any other type of medical disorder. It is hard not to think that the whole concept of 'untreatability' reflects both the personality disordered patient's projected hopelessness about his condition; and a hostility in psychiatric professionals towards those patients who are not grateful to us, or who do not make us feel good by getting better quicker. In this paper, the concept of treatability is analysed in a little more detail; as to how and why it is used in relation to personality disorder.

They murmured, as they took their fees
'There is no cure for this disease'.

Hilaire Belloc

[*] Originally published in *Advances in Psychiatric Treatment*, 7, 6, 407–416. Reprinted here by permission of The Royal College of Psychiatrists.

Treatability is a confused and confusing concept in psychiatry. In its legal sense, it is a measure that limits the involuntary admission of patients with some particular types of mental disorder. The legal term itself has generated considerable discussion and dissent (e.g. Mawson, 1983; Grounds, 1987), and the Government's White Paper on reforming mental health legislation in England and Wales proposes to abolish it (Department of Health, 2000). It is, however, a word that also has medical significance. Its use has given rise to another equally confusing concept, 'untreatability'. This article looks at this concept in more detail and examines its strengths and limitations in relation to personality disorder. It argues that treatability is linked to resources and training, as well as psychopathology, and that different understandings of personality disorder may alter ideas about treatability. This discussion is relevant in the light of the White Paper's proposals and relates also to the Government's proposals for managing dangerous individuals with personality disorder (Home Office, 1999). The discussion, however, focuses on 'treatability' as a clinical term, and does not consider the legal aspects in any detail.

PERSONALITY DISORDER: AN ILLNESS?

Box 1 outlines the case of Kieran. Reading this clinical vignette, we might ask, is Kieran ill? And if not, why not? In this article, I will set out some of the arguments about the nosological status of personality disorder in terms of illness and disease.

The debate about personality disorder's status as a mental illness needs to be seen in the context of the more general debate about the extent to which mental distress of any sort can be understood as a disease, illness, disability or disorder. Again, discussions in this area are complicated by the fact that, in English law, 'mental disorder' and 'mental illness' are terms that have specific legal meanings in addition to a more general clinical usage.

DESCRIPTIVE VS. NORMATIVE ACCOUNTS OF DISORDERS

The status of mental disorder as illness or disease is still a potent source of debate (for a review, see Fulford, 1989; see also Box 2). Much of the debate has centred around the tension between what are called descriptive and normative accounts. Descriptive accounts of disorders claim that it is possible to describe and classify a disease and/or illness without making some sort of value (or normative) judgement about the concept. Normative accounts claim the reverse: that there is no 'objective' account of disorders that does not contain

---

Box 1 Clinical vignette

Kieran is a young man, who has been self-harming for several years, since his late-teens. He regularly presents at different casualty departments around the country, always using different names and giving different accounts of himself. He is also regularly in trouble with the criminal justice system for shoplifting. He attends outpatient appointments to see his psychiatrist and takes prescribed antidepressant medication. Recently, his self-harming behaviour has been getting much worse, and his family want him to be admitted to hospital, involuntarily if necessary. The general practitioner and approved social worker are unsure how best to proceed, as the consultant psychiatrist refuses to admit Kieran, saying: 'He's not ill, he's got a personality disorder.'

---

some reference to an established value or norm. Theorists such as Boorse (1975) have argued that the term 'disease' describes the pathological processes that then give rise to 'illness' as experienced by the patient. 'Diseases' then are those processes that can be described objectively, whereas 'illness' is more subjective, and necessarily involves a normative (value judgement) component.

BIOLOGICAL DISADVANTAGE

This distinction between disease and illness has been highly influential, although still leaving room for debate; for example, whether, and to what extent, the terms 'illness' and 'disease' may actually be synonymous. The arguments become even more complex when applied to mental disorders. Most readers will be familiar with claims that all diagnosis of mental disorder is really 'only' or 'just' a type of value judgement (an argument put most forcefully by Thomas Szasz). Boorse (1975) himself suggested that, on this account, it is difficult for any mental disorder to be a disease, although there might be many mental illnesses. Scadding (1988) argued that there may be different overlapping accounts of diseases (syndromal, pathological or aetiological), but that the key feature of a disease is related to the extent to which it puts a biological organism at 'biological disadvantage'. This notion of biological disadvantage has been used to justify the claim that mental disorder has equal disease status with physical disorder (e.g. Kendell, 1975).

HARMFUL DYSFUNCTION

Wakefield (1992) has argued that it may be helpful to understand mental disorder as 'harmful dysfunction': a combination of a normative illness account and a descriptive account of loss of function, as determined by evolution. Other theorists have argued that the evaluative/normative aspect of diagnosis is an essential feature of both physical and mental disorders (e.g. Fulford, 1989; Engelhardt, 1999), and mental disorders therefore need not be seen as something conceptually different. The fact that value judgements may be part of diagnosis does not mean that there cannot be agreement between clinicians, or that the disorder is less 'real' (Fulford, 2000).

Box 2 Concepts of health disorders

The following are much debated:

  Illness: subjective experience, includes suffering?

  Disease: the pathological processes underlying illness?

  Dysfunction: failure of normal action?

  Disability: a chronic dysfunctional state?

  Disorder: all of the above?

  Relevance of statistical deviance from norms?

NEGATIVELY EVALUATED BEHAVIOUR

Few of these theorists have applied their analysis to personality disorder. For-malised diagnostic criteria, such as the DSM or ICD, have tended to equate symptoms with negatively evaluated behaviours, such as deliberate self-harm or violence to others. This causes conceptual problems because usual accounts of illness, and illness behaviour, define 'symptoms' as actions or experiences that are not willed, desired or chosen by the patient. However, negatively evaluated behaviour is so evaluated precisely because it is perceived to be chosen or willed by the patient, and behaviours or experiences that are willed or chosen are not symptoms.

Behaviours and symptoms cannot always be synonymous, especially in the domain of negatively evaluated behaviour. Therefore a theoretical approach that classifies or understands personality disorder in terms of behaviour leads to two problems. Either any negatively evaluated behaviour, such as self-harm or violence to others, is seen as actually willed 'badness' (leaving aside for a moment what that might mean), and people with personality disorders are equated with people who behave badly; or it may be argued that 'bad' behaviour is not a feature of illness, and therefore people with personality disorder are not ill (e.g. Eldergill, 1999).

There are real philosophical objections, and empirical difficulties, with both positions. One principal objection is that 'bad' behaviour can be associated (but is not synonymous) with some types of mental illness, as demonstrated by the risk and mental disorder literature. Another objection is the albeit limited evidence that some aspects of 'bad' behaviour have a neurological substrate, and may be influenced by genes for arousal and affect control; whether this would be sufficient to justify the definition of personality disorder as an 'illness' is a moot point in itself.

Focusing on negatively evaluated behaviours as symptoms distracts attention from other ways of conceptualising 'personality disorder'. More recent accounts (including DSM-IV; American Psychiatric Association, 1994) emphasise the significant failure of interpersonal functioning seen in personality disorder, which arises as a result of a variety of psychological deficits (Blackburn, 1998). Some psychiatrists have argued strongly that personality disorder is an illness on the grounds of resulting biological disadvantage to the individual (Gunn, 1992, 1999). Other clinicians have noted the degree of subjective suffering experienced by patients with personality disorder (Norton, 1996), which would normally be understood as a necessary (although not sufficient) feature of an illness. Many studies have noted that patients with personality disorder frequently also suffer from other concurrent mental illnesses, such as anxiety, mood disorders and schizophrenia. Taylor (1999) has argued that one can claim personality to be an illness in so far as it reduces individual variance; people with personality disorder are more like each other than not.

THE SICKNESS ROLE

A possible solution to the problems described above may lie in Talcott Parsons' notion of the 'sickness role'. People who are ill are expected to avoid behaving in ways that exacerbate their condition, accept the idea that they need help, have the desire to get better and seek competent help to do so (Mechanic, 1978). However, many people with personality disorders, although claiming to be ill and in need, do not behave in the ways expected of a sick person. Perhaps we could understand this failure to fulfil sick role expectations as a type of psychological disability – an incapacity to obtain care effectively – which would undoubtedly convey a biological disadvantage in the long term.

DISABILITY

Fulford (1989) has argued that it might be helpful to understand personality disorders as disabilities, rather than illnesses. Accounts of disability usually emphasise the chronic nature of the patient's problems; they also emphasise the interpersonal aspects of function and dysfunction for people with disabilities. Some readers may remember an advertising campaign for people with disabilities that ran the slogan 'Our biggest handicap is other people's attitudes'. Such an interpersonal view is found in American legal definitions of disability (Silver, 1999) and it may be a useful way to understand the difficulties faced by people with disability in terms of making choices and being agents of their own destiny (Agich, 1993).

IS PERSONALITY DISORDER AN ILLNESS?

The status of personality disorder as an illness therefore remains contentious, especially while it is defined simply in terms of behaviour. Scadding (1988) has argued that most accounts of mental disorder are at a syndromal, or symptom level, and that illness claims are stronger when there is an aetiological account. Aetiological models have only recently been developed for personality disorder. These models draw on research from longitudinal follow-up studies of child development, and the impact of traumatic events of the personality functioning of adults. Both retrospective and longitudinal studies suggest that early childhood adversity is a potent risk factor for the development of a personality disorder in adulthood (Modestin et al., 1998; Johnson et al., 1999). Studies of the effects of exposure in adulthood to traumatic and frightening events also indicate that such events may cause change and damage to the personality (as found in the diagnosis of 'enduring personality change after trauma', defined in ICD-10; World Health Organization, 1992).

If external events in both childhood and adulthood can shape adult personality functioning, then it is possible to understand personality disorder as an acquired, rather than an innate, condition. Although this argument will not deal with all the conceptual difficulties surrounding the disease/illness status of personality disorder, it does at least challenge the view that some people are just 'born' with personality disorder – a sort of psychiatric version of St Augustine's notion of original sin.

Box 3 Personality disorder and concepts of health

Is personality disorder:

- an illness (suffering; biological disadvantage)?

- a pejorative label, used to describe 'bad' behaviour?

- caused by a disease process (amygdala dysfunction, abnormal arousal patterns)?

- acquired as a result of adverse or traumatic environmental experience?

- another term for 'deviant' or 'criminal', and nothing to do with health?

- a complex manifestation of multiple disabilities?

- all/none/some of the above?

TREATMENT AND TREATABILITY

General medical considerations

I want now to think about what it means to be able to treat a disorder, any clinical disorder. Treatments may have different purposes, not all of which aim at cure. Several recent court judgements about treatments for physical diseases have made it clear that 'treatment' includes a broad range of interventions aimed at bringing about a beneficial outcome; and this benefit may be defined as change of symptoms, enhancement of quality of life or prevention of further damage.

Seven-factor model of treatability

What makes a physical condition treatable? I would like to suggest that treatability is a function of seven factors operating simultaneously (Box 4). No one factor will determine a condition's treatability and, especially, its 'untreatability'. We can apply this model to any disorder. I will take as an example the treatment of cancer, partly because it is a disorder that sometimes attracts fear and stigma as well as sympathy, and partly because the term 'un-treatable' is a term of significance for cancer patients and their families.

The type of cancer is a crucial factor in looking at treatability and prognosis, since it is well established that different types may be more or less treatable. The treatability of the cancer will depend on its anatomical context

---

Box 4 The seven-factor model of treatability

1 The nature and severity of pathology: site, histology, grade.

2 The involvement of other bodily systems: spread, impact on function.

3 The patient's previous health, comorbidity, risk factors.

4 The timing of intervention: diagnosis, early/late identification, action.

5 The experience and availability of staff.

6 Availability of specialist units for special conditions.

7 State of knowledge; cultural attitudes.

(site) and nature (e.g. histological grading, differentiation). The spread of the cancer affects its treatability – more extensive spread may make some types of treatment more difficult. Premorbid health is a relevant factor in assessing treatability, in so far as it reveals risk and resilience factors that may affect the course of the disorder.

The timing of any treatment for cancer influences treatability, given that there is evidence supporting early rather than late intervention. This in turn relates to the process of diagnosis and identification of the problem. In many cases, treatment is delayed, either because symptoms are not understood as being those of cancer, or because symptoms are thought to be caused by another condition. Such uncertainty about identification of symptoms and diagnosis can lead to delay, which in turn affects treatment response.

Once detected, treatability is affected by the availability of specialists familiar with the specific problems posed by different sorts of cancer. There is good evidence, for example, that the treatability (and prognosis) of breast cancer is influenced by the availability of specialist breast cancer surgeons. Such specialists are backed up by specialist teams, with access to specialist facilities and equipment. Such specialist treatment rarely provides a cure for the cancer; nevertheless, therapy is still offered that improves quality of life and offers support to those who care for and support the patient.

Lastly, most cancers are more treatable now than 10 or 15 years ago: better understanding of the different conditions, their course and nature have offered improved ways of offering treatment. Very few cancer treatments, especially for severe conditions, have been exposed to randomised controlled trials to prove their efficacy; yet they are used clinically to good effect. It is also worth considering the strong ethical arguments against carrying out such trials.

Application of the seven-factor model to personality disorder

I hope it will already be apparent that there are parallels between the treatment of cancer and the treatment of personality disorder. In relation to diagnosis, a simple statement of 'personality disorder' is likely to be misleading. Most individuals can be diagnosed as having more than one personality disorder, indicating a range of difficulties. The predominant type is relevant, however, because different interventions may be indicated for different types of personality disorder (Davidson, 2001). The evidence base for treatment of personality disorder generally is still limited, but this concern is more a feature of Factor 7 (i.e. state of scientific knowledge) than a characteristic of the disorder itself. It is also worth remembering that 20 or 30 years ago, 'cancer' was also treated as a somewhat unitary diagnostic identity with a gloomy prognosis.

Factor 1: Nature and severity

Whatever the limitations of the current typologies, it is clear that not all personality disorders are the same. It is also clear that there are degrees of severity; the term 'severe personality disorder' has been in usage for over 30 years (e.g. Craft *et al.*, 1964; Department of Health/Home Office, 1986; Tyrer and Johnson, 1996) and is not simply a contemporary political invention. Equally, it is likely that there are both 'mild' and 'moderate' degrees of personality disorder, characterised by significant interpersonal dysfunction, but without the more extreme behavioural manifestations. These conditions may be made worse by the presence of other factors, such as Axis I disorders, or new stressors. Such a dimensional approach provides a better description of the clinical complexities observed in practice. The evidence to date suggests that mild and moderate severe personality disorders are treatable with appropriate therapeutic interventions (Fonagy and Roth, 1996; Lees *et al.*, 1999).

Factor 2: Degree of spread

In the case of personality disorder, 'spread' would be represented by the patient's degree of involvement in other psychological, health and social systems and the impact on functioning in different areas of their life (Remington and Tyrer, 1979). Different degrees of involvement with different systems could be seen as a measure of severity; that is, an individual who has been involved with health, social and criminal justice systems as a result of a personality disorder is likely to be less treatable than one who has been involved only with health care providers. Severity may also be indicated by the frequency, variety and harmfulness of any risk behaviours. Such an approach is supported by the literature on mental disorder and risk, which indicates that risk factors are additive (Swanson, 1994). The emphasis is on understanding the behaviours as manifestations of interpersonal dysfunction, just as abnormal gait may be a behavioural manifestation of metastatic disease.

Factor 3: Comorbidity

The treatability of any disorder is likely to be reduced when there is comorbidity with other disorders. This is frequently the case for personality disorder, where comorbidity with mood disorders and substance misuse are especially common. Treatability is also likely to be affected by developmental history, and the presence of risk and resilience factors. For example, most therapists assessing the treatability of personality disorder will look at the history of interpersonal relating from early childhood, arguing that treatment is more likely to be successful if there is any history of a positive attachment to another person.

Factor 4: Identification, diagnosis and timing

Clearly, personality disorder will be not be 'treatable' if it is not identified as a disorder: hence the relevance of the illness debate discussed above. There are empirical questions to be answered here: if two individuals with similar presentations are assessed, and both are understood as having a personality disorder but only one is treated, what difference does that make to subsequent treatability? Do early interventions prevent later pathology? Ongoing studies of adolescents with personality disorder may provide information about this: what is established is that patients with personality disorder are unpopular and rejected by services (Appleby and Lewis, 1988). The point here is whether the process of rejection, and failure to identify pathology, itself affects the treatability of the condition, so that each negative encounter makes the condition worse.

Factors 5 and 6: Specialist staff and facilities

Factors 5 and 6 relate to the provision of specialist staff and facilities. Clinicians who either do not accept personality disorder as a pathological condition, or who have no experience in treating the condition even if they do, may well be justified in saying that personality disorder is untreatable by them or in their units. The issue here is that factors outside the patient's condition may make them untreatable, rather than some innate feature of their condition. Given what we know about the adverse early childhood experience in personality disorder and the difficulties in constructive help-seeking that is often a feature, it is very unlikely that many individuals with personality disorders will be 'treatable' in facilities that require them to be obedient, compliant, passive and grateful.

A claim that treatability may be a function of service availability is further supported by evidence that where specialist help is provided, both in terms of staff and facilities, therapeutic benefits are possible in some types of personality disorder (Dolan *et al.*, 1996; Bateman and Fonagy, 1999; Lees *et al.*, 1999; Perry *et al.*, 1999). The case is then no different from that of some types of cancer, where effective therapeutic interventions will only be offered by some specialist units. No one would argue that conditions such as cancer are globally 'untreatable', only that treatment and treatability may be limited by access to and availability of trained staff.

Availability of specialist staff and services raises the question of resource allocation in the treatment of personality disorder. It is not possible to quantify exactly the resources needed, although some estimate might be made based on primary care prevalence figures and usage of services at all levels. Some evidence exists that demonstrates that where specialist therapy is offered and completed, the costs involved are offset by the subsequent reduction of service usage by patients with personality disorder (Dolan *et al.*, 1996). Resource allocation in medicine generally is a complex ethical decision-making process. To date, allocation of resources for the treatment of mental disorders has favoured the needs of those with chronic psychotic disorders, who may be seen as more deserving, more conventionally 'ill' and easier to treat with medication that is cheap. Resources for the treatment of personality disorder tend to become available when required as a means of controlling violence to third parties, which reinforces the conflation of a personality disorder diagnosis with violence. Even in the context of violence, resources are not concentrated on those patients with personality disorder who are violent to partners or children, but rather on the minority who are more generally violent, often in bizarre ways.

Factor 7: Scientific knowledge and cultural attitudes
Factor 7 involves the state of scientific knowledge, and the influence of both that evidence base and cultural attitudes on treatability of personality disorder.

There has been a real increase in the scientific study of personality disorder over the past 10 years (Gunn, 1999), but there is still extensive empirical ground to make up. Basic knowledge about the natural history, course and prognosis are still lacking – a review published 10 years ago raises many questions to which there are still no answers (Tyrer *et al.*, 1991). Given such a lack of evidence, it seems illogical (not to say irrational) to state categorically that personality disorder is not an illness because it does not have an established course or prognosis (Ferguson and Milton, 2000).

An evidenced-based position supports two claims about personality disorder that are important in considering treatability. First, the evidence that personality disorder may in part be an acquired condition justifies clinicians taking time to think in more complex ways about individuals with personality disorders. Second, there is good evidence that some types of personality disorder, probably of mild-to-moderate severity, do respond to some types of treatment – usually a combination of psychological and pharmacological interventions delivered by clinical teams with experience and training. There is therefore no justification for global assertions that personality disorder is untreatable – a view that is still taught to trainees, asserted in journals and stated as expert evidence in court.

There is equally no evidence that all personality disorders would be treatable if only the clinician's attitude were right and there were enough facilities. A grandiose attitude to the management of personality disorder may be as damaging as a nihilistic one (Cawthra, 2000). Just as in other medical domains, there are likely to be many cases where the damage is so great, and the interpersonal systems failure so profound, that no treatment is going to bring about improvement for the individual. To date, we have no evidence that therapies are available that can ameliorate severe personality disorder which gives rise to significant harm to self and others. However, people with severe personality disorders arguably may still require interventions that are therapeutic, or at least not anti-therapeutic. Their needs resemble those cases in palliative care where interventions are still offered, if only in terms of a supportive environment and support for staff who are involved in the daily management of such cases. Alternatively, if one understood these people as cases of severe disability (picking up Fulford's argument), therapeutic interventions could be aimed at damage limitation, quality of life issues and the management of despair and grief at what has been lost and cannot be repaired.

CONCLUSIONS

> If you can meet with triumph and disaster, and treat those two impostors
> just the same.

> Rudyard Kipling

My argument here is that the assessment of treatability of personality disorder
is a complex process, which is multifactorial and operational in nature. The
approach outlined above is clearly only a preliminary account, which could be
further developed. Such an approach might generate ways of rating treatability,
which could then be assessed empirically for validity and reliability in different
clinical settings.

I have outlined some of the factors I consider to be central to providing a
good quality assessment of treatability; no doubt there are others that will be
relevant. For example, I have not discussed the question of repeat assessment,
which would take account of both temporal change and the interpersonal
nature of the dysfunction to be assessed. One-off assessments alone may be
highly unreliable (Bass and Murphy, 1995). Motivation is important, since
individuals with personality disorder (like any other patient group) may also be
more or less willing to get engaged in treatment, depending on circumstances.
Paradoxically, a time of crisis may not be the best time to start some types of
treatment; different treatments may be more or less appropriate at different
times.

I will close by thinking briefly about the implications of this discussion for
services. The key message is that not all patients with personality disorder are
the same. Different psychiatric services are likely to meet different types of personality disorder, of different levels of severity, and may therefore need to
develop different therapeutic approaches. Clearly, specialist services for personality disorder will be able to offer interventions that cannot be offered in
primary care; however, it may be a mistake to generalise from those specialist
services to less specialist general ones.

Three different service providers may have specific roles to play. Psychotherapy services will be important providers, not just of highly specialised
services such as out-patient and in-patient therapeutic communities, but also as
sources of advice, consultation and supervision to adult mental health and
primary care (NHS Executive, 1996). Child and adolescent services will be
involved with young people whose personality disorder may be more amenable
to treatment (which can be empirically studied); they will also see a group of
people with personality disorders who are dangerous only to their children.
Such individuals arguably also suffer from severe and dangerous personality

disorder, but are rarely offered any sort of intervention. Lastly, secure forensic services will probably see people with the most severe and dangerous personality disorders. They will therefore need additional resources in terms of psychological therapists, both medical and non-medical, of all theoretical schools. This is especially necessary in order to develop therapeutic strategies for managing men and women who may have to reside in some sort of secure care for the rest of their lives. As my late and much missed predecessor, Murray Cox, once said: 'If no one ever left Broadmoor, you would need more staff not less.'

We need to be developing better education and training for junior medical staff and other members of multi-disciplinary teams managing people with personality disorder. Provision of staff education and support, which helps staff to understand the impact of working with patients with personality disorder, makes therapeutic interventions more possible (Norton, 1996) and is valued by staff (Krawitz and RREAL, 2001). This is not to say that all the problems will vanish, only that they may be more manageable.

Personality disorder still presents considerable conceptual and therapeutic challenges. We still struggle with defining it, diagnosing it and dealing with its more destructive behavioural manifestations. As the behaviours become more dangerous and frightening to others, so we have seen that sections of the public, including government, hope that psychiatry can offer something that will make people not just feel better, but behave better. The clinician/researcher who could do such a thing might get a Nobel Prize (and make a lot of money). The more likely course for psychiatrists is that we will continue to have to manage very difficult people with scarce resources; and somehow avoid falling into either angry despair or mindless optimism. As Kipling suggests, 'triumph' and 'disaster' may both be psychological impostors.

Disclaimer

Although the facts are clinically accurate, Kieran's case is fictitious and does not represent any real patient, alive or dead.

REFERENCES

Agich, G. (1993) *Autonomy in Long-Term Care.* Oxford: Oxford University Press.

American Psychiatric Association. (1994) *Diagnostic and Statistical Manual of Mental Disorders* (4th ed.) (DSM-IV). Washington, DC: APA.

Appleby, L. and Lewis, G. (1988) Personality disorder: the patients psychiatrists dislike. *British Journal of Psychiatry*, 153, 44–49.

Bass, C. and Murphy, M. (1995) Somatoform and personality disorders: Syndromal comorbidity and overlapping developmental pathways. *Journal of Psychosomatic Research*, 39, 403–427.

Bateman, A. and Fonagy, P. (1999) Treatment of borderline personality disorder. *American Journal of Psychiatry*, 156,1563–1568.

Blackburn, R. (1998) 'Psychopathy and the contribution of personality to violence.' In T. Millon, E. Simonson, M. Birket-Smith *et al.*, eds. *Psychopathy: Antisocial, Criminal and Violent Behaviour.* London: Guilford Press. p.50–68.

Boorse, C. (1975) On the distinction between illness and disease. *Philosophy and Public Affairs*, 5, 49–68. Reprinted in J. Lindemann Nelson and H. Lindemann Nelson, H. eds. (1999) *Meaning and Medicine: A Reader in the Philosophy of Health Care.* London: Routledge. p.16–27.

Cawthra, R. (2000) Commentary on recent developments in borderline personality disorder. *Advances in Psychiatric Treatment*, 6, 217–218.

Craft, M., Stephenson, G. and Granger, C. (1964) The relationship between severity of personality disorder and certain adverse childhood influences. *British Journal of Psychiatry*, 110, 392–396.

Davidson, S. (2002) The principles of managing patients with personality disorder. *Advances in Psychiatric Treatment*, 8, 1–9.

Department of Health, (2000) *Reforming the Mental Health Act: Part II: High Risk Patients.* Cm 5016-2. London: Department of Health.

Department of Health/Home Office, (1986) *Offenders Suffering from Psychopathic Disorder.* Joint Consultation Paper: London: HMSO.

Dolan, B.M., Warren, F.M., Menzies, D., *et al.* (1996) Cost-offset following specialist treatment of severe personality disorders. *Psychiatric Bulletin*, 20, 413–417.

Eldergill, A. (1999) Psychopathy, the law and individual rights. *Princeton University Law Journal*, III, 1–30.

Engelhardt, T. (1999) 'The disease of masturbation: value and the concept of disease.' In J. Lindemann Nelson and H. Lindemann Nelson, eds. *Meaning and Medicine: A Reader in the Philosophy of Health Care.* London: Routledge. p.5–15.

Ferguson, B. and Milton, J. (2000) Editorial. *Irish Journal of Psychological Medicine*, 17, 3–4.

Fonagy, P. and Roth, P. (1996) *What Works for Whom?* London: Sage.

Fulford, K.W. (1989) *Moral Theory and Medical Practice.* Cambridge: Cambridge University Press.

Fulford, K.W. (2000) 'Disordered minds, diseased brains and real people.' In C. Heginbotham, ed. *Philosophy, Psychiatry and Psychopathy: Personal Identity in Mental Disorder.* Aldershot: Ashgate Publishing. p.47–75.

Grounds, A. (1987) Detention of 'psychopathic disorder' patients in special hospitals. Critical issues. *British Journal of Psychiatry*, 151, 474–478.

Gunn, J. (1992) Personality disorders and forensic psychiatry. *Criminal Behaviour and Mental Health*, 2, 202–211.

Gunn, J. (1999) 'Written evidence.' In *Department of Health Report of the Committee of Enquiry into the Personality Disorder Unit, Ashworth Special Hospital. Vol. II: Expert Evidence on Personality Disorder*, p.207. Cm 4195. London: Stationery Office.

Home Office/Department of Health, (1999) *Managing Dangerous People with Severe Personality Disorder: Proposals for Policy Development.* London: Home Office/ Department of Health.

Johnson, J., Cohen, P., Brown, J., *et al.* (1999) Childhood maltreatment increases risk for personality disorders during early adulthood. *Archives of General Psychiatry*, 56, 600–606.

Kendell, R. (1975) The concept of disease and its implications for psychiatry. *British Journal of Psychiatry*, 127, 305–315.

Krawitz, R. and RREAL (Resource Team for Borderline Syndrome), (2001) Borderline personality disorder: foundation training for public mental health clinicians. *Australasian Psychiatry*, 9, 25–28.

Lees, J., Manning, N. and Rawlings, B. (1999) *Therapeutic Community Effectiveness*. NHS Centre Reviews and Dissemination, Report 17. York: University of York.

Mawson, D. (1983) 'Psychopaths' in special hospitals. *Psychiatric Bulletin*, 7, 178–181.

Mechanic, D. (1978) *Medical Sociology* (2nd ed). New York: Free Press.

Modestin, J., Oberson, B. and Erni, T. (1998) Possible antecedents of DSM-III-R personality disorders. *Acta Psychiatric Scandinavia*, 97, 260–266.

NHS Executive, (1996) *Review of Psychotherapy Services*. London: Department of Health.

Norton, K. (1996) Management of difficult personality disorder patients. *Advances in Psychiatric Treatment*, 2, 202–210.

Perry, J.C., Banon, E. and Ianni, F. (1999) Effectiveness of psychotherapy for personality disorders. *American Journal of Psychiatry*, 156, 1312–1321.

Remington, M. and Tyrer, P. (1979) The social functioning schedule – a brief semi-structured interview. *Social Psychiatry*, 14, 151–157.

Scadding, J. (1988) Health and disease: What can medicine do for philosophy? *Journal of Medical Ethics*, 14, 118–124.

Silver, A. (1999) '(In)Equality, (Ab)Normality and the Americans with Disabilities Act.' In J. Lindemann Nelson and H. Lindemann Nelson, eds. *Meaning and Medicine: A Reader in the Philosophy of Health Care*. London: Routledge. p.28–37.

Swanson, J. (1994) 'Mental disorder, substance abuse, and community violence: an epidemiological approach.' In J. Monahan and H. Steadman, eds. *Mental Disorder and Violence*. Chicago: University of Chicago Press. p.101–136.

Taylor, P.J. (1999) 'Written evidence.' In *Department of Health Report of the Committee of Enquiry into the Personality Disorder Unit, Ashworth Special Hospital. Vol. II: Expert Evidence on Personality Disorder*, p.489. Cm 4195. London: Stationery Office.

Tyrer, P. and Johnson, T. (1996) Establishing the severity of personality disorder. *American Journal of Psychiatry*, 153, 593–597.

Tyrer, P., Casey, P. and Ferguson, B. (1991) Personality disorder in perspective. *British Journal of Psychiatry*, 159, 463–471.

Wakefield, J. (1992) Disorder as harmful dysfunction: a conceptual critique of DSM-III-R's definition of mental disorder. *Psychological Review*, 99, 232–247.

World Health Organisation, (1992) *International Classification of Mental and Behavioural Disorders* (ICD-10) Geneva: WHO.

12

Management of Difficult Personality Disorder Patients[*]

Kingsley Norton
1996

· ·

Editors' reflections

This is another paper from Kingsley Norton; this time exploring how therapy can be problematic for both patients with personality disorders and their therapists. Treatment can be 'arduous' if we do not distinguish the interpersonal problems from the personality problem itself, that is if we do not distinguish between the problem, and the defence against the problem. He makes reference to the value of coordinated therapies in the treatment of personality disorder, and the appropriate prescription of medication. He also makes use of attachment theory as a paradigm for understanding personality pathology.

· ·

INTRODUCTION

> ...Therapy often becomes part of the problem rather than vice versa.
> (George Lockwood, 1992)

Ten per cent of the general adult population have a diagnosable personality disorder (Zimmerman and Coryell, 1990) and in 4% this is clinically severe (Tyrer, 1988). The clinical management of such patients may be difficult.

---

[*] Originally published in *Advances in Psychiatric Treatment*, 2, 202–210. Reprinted here by permission of The Royal College of Psychiatrists.

However, much clinical difficulty is generated by interpersonal aspects deriving from the particular interaction of the patient and psychiatrist involved and the respective roles they play.

It is important, therefore, to distinguish between the clinical problem proper and those aspects of the personal interaction of patient and psychiatrist which may unhelpfully (including via stigmatic labelling) contribute to the complexity of the case, further complicating the clinical management of it (Norton and Smith, 1994). This is because interpersonal issues often become so prominent, in clinical transactions with personality disordered patients, that they make it impossible to achieve or maintain an ordinary clinical focus which could identify relevant and achievable goals of treatment.

The psychiatrist can be side-tracked by such interpersonal aspects but recognising this may be problematic, since the distraction from a proper clinical focus may be subtle and is not necessarily negative in quality. There may be an inappropriately positive interpersonal influence, at least initially (Yeomans, 1993). Whether the distraction is positive or negative, what is missing is an appropriate level of mutual respect and trust, so vital for carrying out the professional level clinical tasks. Too often the psychiatrist mistakenly takes its existence for granted.

The aim of this paper is to identify some of the common pitfalls in the clinical management of personality disordered patients, indicating how they can be avoided or otherwise dealt with, so making treatment less arduous.

DIAGNOSIS AND ENGAGEMENT

An unreliable or invalid diagnosis of personality disorder often reflects poor diagnostic technique, as much as it reflects inadequate definitions or inaccurate measures of personality disorder. Thus, sometimes there appears to be ignorance of the need to engage the personality disordered individual, as a patient, rather than to take for granted their ability to perform the role of patient successfully. Without adequate engagement, it is not possible to elicit an accurate history or mental state examination and so on, hence no diagnosis is reliable.

Diagnostic subcategories

The validity of subcategories of personality disorder is uncertain and some prefer to view personality disorder as a unitary syndrome (Coid, 1989), a view given support by the presence of more than one personality disorder subtype diagnosis in individual patients (Zimmerman *et al.*, 1991). The number of personality disorder subtype diagnoses, per personality disordered patient, is associated with the particular psychiatric setting (see Dolan *et al.*, 1995), the highest numbers being recorded in the most secure in-patient settings, wherein are experienced some of the greatest clinical management problems. In such settings it may be the exception, rather than the rule, to find single subcategory personality disorder diagnosis. The number of personality disorder subtype diagnoses in an individual patient therefore may be a marker of the severity of the overall personality disorder (Dolan *et al.*, 1995).

In view of the presence of more than one personality disorder subtype in so many personality disordered psychiatric patients, especially in those who present extreme difficulty in their clinical management, personality disorder will be considered here as a unitary syndrome.

Box 1 Clinical difficulty and PD patients

(1) PD is not in itself inherently untreatable.

(2) PD patients can be difficult to manage because of:

   (i)   Difficulties in diagnosing PD or a missed diagnosis of PD.

   (ii) Coexistence of a symptom disorder that complicates the treatment of PD and vice versa.

(3) Some PD patients cannot or will not play their complementary role as patients.

(4) Interpersonal problems between the psychiatrist and PD patient, arising out of (2) or (3), become the focus of the clinical encounter, thereby supplanting relevant clinical tasks and complicating treatment.

The patient's role

Initially, many with personality disorder who come into contact with psychiatrists are not meaningfully 'patients', in the sense of having a capacity to present a complaint or symptom with the expectation that appropriate professional treatment or help will be forthcoming. Their non-verbal and sometimes their verbal behaviour says: 'Here I am! I've done my bit. Now it's your turn. What are you going to do about it (me)?'

Mr Adams was smoking a cigarette as he entered the consulting room. The consultant psychiatrist had initially interviewed him the previous week, making a diagnosis of generalised anxiety disorder and personality disorder. He now indicated the discreet 'No Smoking' sign situated on the desk. Apparently not heeding this non-verbal request to extinguish the cigarette, Mr Adams continued to inhale. Indeed, he put the cigarette up to his lips and then removed it in an ostentatious manner. All the time he kept his eyes fixed on the consultant. The latter, attempting to meet Mr Adams' steady gaze, silently fumed! After a short while, and no longer able to contain his impatience with what he perceived to be Mr Adams' contemptuous silence, he blurted out, 'Really, Mr Adams, I must ask you to show more consideration for other people and to refrain from smoking'. He then added, with a hint of remorse, 'In any case, it's a very bad habit'.

The consultant later confided to a colleague that he had regretted this outburst, albeit controlled, not least because Mr Adams had, in response, silently stood up and left the room, quietly closing the door behind him. He subsequently failed further appointments that were sent to him.

The first clinical task is thus to aim to ensure that the patient is engaged as a patient. Engagement entails the successful establishment of a collaborative clinical enterprise between psychiatrist and personality disordered individual, resulting in the negotiating of more or less clear and relevant goals relating to diagnosis and treatment. In the above example, the consultant had thought he had successfully engaged Mr Adams at their first interview and he believed there was sufficient trust and respect to permit him his non-verbal request to the patient. He was not aware that he would again have to prove his credit-worthiness, in terms of trust and respect, and could not take such aspects for granted at the second interview.

Obstacles to engagement

There are many obstacles to engagement, yet the development of a therapeutic alliance with the patient is essential as a vehicle of change (Horwitz, 1974; Frank, 1991). Some personality disordered individuals have totally unrealistic expectations of professionals (too high, too low or constantly oscillating between the two extremes) and so will make inappropriate or unrealistic demands. Disabusing them of their misapprehension or educating them about what is realistically available is crucial but it is often experienced as patronising or humiliating and the professional relationship may break down under the burden of the resulting disagreement, anger or disappointment. Failure to engage and maintain a therapeutic alliance (as with Mr Adams) only serves to reinforce the patient's basic mistrust of professionals and the psychiatrist's notion of the difficulty and untreatability of the patient.

Some personality disordered individuals, by virtue of their style of presentation, impel or seduce professionals into attempting to offer more than is realistically available. Such a temptation for the psychiatrist to be 'too good' or 'too powerful', which is often a reaction to the patient's unrealistically high expectations and the former's unwillingness to state limits that might disappoint or frustrate the patient, needs to be avoided (Yeomans, 1993).

INSECURE AND DISORGANISED ATTACHMENTS

The past

Personality disordered patients' basic and pervasive mistrust stems from neglectful and/or abusive childhoods during which parents (or their substitute adults) abused their authority, avoided their parental responsibilities or were highly inconsistent in attitude or behaviour towards their children, many parents being personality disordered themselves (Norton and Dolan, 1995b). The patients' formative years are thus scarred by insecure and disorganised attachments. As a result, their internal working models, influencing their later expectations of others and their styles of relating to them, reflect this (Bowlby, 1973).

Many personality disordered patients thus expect professionals to fail them (as did their parents) even though, usually secretly, they crave an individual who could meet their every need. In the face of this, psychiatrists often feel as if they cannot succeed. If psychiatrists only reinforce part of the patient's view – that no reliable help is available – then they fail the secret view (against all odds and previous experience) that there exists someone who will help responsibly and not abuse their authority. However, any help which is provided is often perceived as insufficient. Falling so far short of the idealised 'perfect help', it can cause further pain and disappointment. As a consequence, the psychiatrist may feel 'damned if he does and damned if he does not treat'.

Patients' lack of familiarity with secure attachments and their ambivalence towards the psychiatrist and treatment therefore need to be assumed and addressed directly, as part of the (ongoing) task of engagement and the forging of a therapeutic alliance.

Box 2 Engaging the PD individual as a patient

(1) The PD patient's capacity to engage in treatment should not be assumed.

(2) Engagement is the result of an active and collaborative endeavour between psychiatrist and patient.

(3) Without adequate engagement the quality and reliability of assessment information is impaired leading to diagnostic and treatment difficulties.

(4) Commonly encountered obstacles to engagement include the patient's:

(i)   Unrealistic expectations of treatment;

(ii) Basic mistrust in professionals;

(iii) Ambivalence about seeking and receiving help.

The present

In-patient staff, particularly, experience difficulties in providing care of consistently high quality in the face of the personality disordered patient's ambivalent wish for it and their consequent lack of engagement. Inconsistency in the delivery of planned treatments increases with the number of staff or number of different agencies that are involved with it. This results for two main reasons: Covert inter-staff disagreements with the treatment approach, which are either unspoken and/or unresolved; and breakdowns in inter-staff communication or the communication of partial or inaccurate information between staff or between agencies (Stanton and Schwartz, 1954; Main, 1957).

For many patients, the combined thrill and terror of the in-patient chase and capture, followed by enforced sedation and/or seclusion or specialling, represents familiar (albeit insecure) emotional territory. Paradoxically, they are reassured by many, though not all, aspects of it. This frantic mutual activity, however, disallows a novel experience which might impel the patients to question their habitual maladaptive attitudes and behaviour – its cognitive and emotional origins, antecedents, and its consequences. The patients' ingrained behaviour patterns and inflexible responses thus endure (Norton and Dolan, 1995c).

Where physical containment (for example, locked wards; enforced medication) predominates, personality disordered patients survive and function. This is because their existing 'inflexible responses' (part of the definition of personality disorder; WHO, 1992) have been shaped by issues of domination and control in the abusive and/or neglecting experiences received during their childhood and adolescence. In such an in-patient environment, just as in the past, apparent care and respect readily transform, either to punishment or else to a remote professional neutrality perceived by the patient as neglect. Professional care is then viewed as counterfeit and simply as a manipulative or seductive camouflage.

Although simple physical containment can afford personality disordered patients temporary and familiar relief, in the longer term they are left feeling misunderstood, righteously indignant and victimised. Indeed, they can appear to be enveloped by such feelings as if in a welcomed embrace. In the absence of anxiety evoked by an environmental response which is felt by them to be empathic, hence novel, patients do not experience conflict sufficiently within themselves – there is a relative absence of a conflictual internal dialogue. They tend to remain more in conflict with others, mainly staff. Thereby, potentially creative internal conflict is avoided and potentially creative energy is discharged and wasted interpersonally.

The future

If patients are to change their mistrustful attitudes to staff, and to begin to work with them collaboratively, they need to give up their oppositional stance. However, this is only achievable if the staff's response is other than to reinforce such a stance. To facilitate this requires of the staff a capacity to consistently apply a treatment approach (withstanding the destructive aspects of staff disagreements and communication problems), and provide a response to the patients' testing behaviour (often violent and manipulative but sometimes involving seductive or erotic behaviour), which does not simply condemn or condone. Thus, staff are required to strive to remain balanced, not taking sides simply for or against, and to examine the particular situation and its relevance to the patient.

This approach may include reiterating that certain aspects of the patient's behaviour are not acceptable and will not be tolerated but it requires, in addition, a questioning and a quest to understand the antecedents and consequences of the behaviour.

In this way, the patient's behaviour may be both condemned and understood. This is a more complex construction than simply condemning or condoning and it can be communicated to the patient. Through this process,

---

Box 3 Correctable reasons for treatment failure

(1)   Inadequate engagement in treatment.

(2)   Unrealistic treatment expectations and time-frame.

(3)   Inconsistent delivery of treatment due to the involvement of more than one agent or agency, leading to:

    (i)   Covert staff disagreements which are unresolved and/or

    (ii)   Breakdown or other inadequacy in inter-staff communication.

(4)   Undue delay in response to deterioration or improvement in the patient's clinical status.

---

patients can learn to understand that they are perceived by others as more than just their 'behaviour' and that the condemnation of their behaviour is not a total personal attack or annihilation. The aim is to help the patients, in spite of their ambivalence about receiving help and their chronic low self-esteem, to become 'thinkers and feelers' rather than simply 'actors' of maladaptive behaviour (Masterson, 1972).

USING A TREATMENT CONTRACT

Even with personality disordered patients who have not been particularly dangerous or disturbed, clinical transactions with them may be complicated rather than straightforward. Thus the ordinary collaborative goal-directed activity of the clinical encounter (out-patient or in-patient) may require buttressing by the establishment of a treatment contract.

A treatment contract involves formalising the usually implicit agreement, which exists between patient and doctor in a straightforward clinical transaction. If it is established early, before basic mistrust and prior insecure or disorganised attachment patterns are reinforced by the current relationship and interaction, it can serve to anchor an agreement to achieve relevant goals by minimising the influence of destructive or distracting personality 'clashes' between patient and doctor. As a beneficial by-product, the patient may derive enhanced self-esteem, through being enabled to play the role of patient more successfully, and the psychiatrist may gain professional satisfaction.

The treatment contract may usefully involve people from the patient's wider social network, especially where they are likely to be directly affected by the meeting of contractual conditions. It can help to have the patient, staff and, in some cases family and/or friends, as literal co-signatories to the contract (Miller, 1989). The more staff or agencies who are involved, the more urgent is the need to have regular meetings of all concerned, lest inconsistencies in the treatment approach emerge and remain undetected and unremedied.

Establishing a treatment contract is easier said than done. It often entails exploring and changing the patient's basic mistrust; ambivalence about seeking help; low self-esteem; ways of dealing with impulses to injure (self or others); and idiosyncratic obstacles to giving up an immature chemical dependence (on drugs or alcohol) in favour of a more mature dependence on people.

Pitfalls

The most common pitfall is for the treatment contract to be introduced at a time when either or both the psychiatrist and the patient are feeling hostile to one another. Under such circumstances it is not likely to succeed in its stated aims. Hostility, especially where this may have formed part of the psychiatrist's motivation to implement the contract in the first place, must have begun to subside before a treatment contract can be successfully negotiated. Negotiating the contract may require considerable time, tact and diplomacy just when such attributes are in short supply. The patient may experience the psychiatrist as authoritarian or patronising, especially if there is, or has been in the past, compulsory treatment or if contractual conditions are set which the patient cannot meet. If this is the case, the contract is likely to break down even if there has been an apparent initial agreement to it.

> Ms Banks, an in-patient for more than six months, had been compulsorily admitted. The diagnosis was of anorexia nervosa with features of a coexisting affective disorder (including serious suicidal ideation and parasuicidal activity) and an underlying dissocial personality disorder. She made little progress initially and, with staff's mounting anxiety about the unlikelihood of her survival, a treatment contract was established out of desperation and frustration, with little staff confidence that it might help.
>
> The contract stated that Ms Banks would accept a high calorie diet with the aim of achieving a weight increase to a mutually agreed level. Staff agreed to stop their cajoling and coaxing of Ms Banks to eat in return for her agreement to attend and speak in her individual sessions. (She had often found reasons not to attend and had avoided talking in depth.)

To the surprise of the team, Ms Banks began to accept her diet and achieved her contracted target weight. However, she did this without divulging any personal difficulties or other information about herself. The staff treating her were grateful that compliance with re-feeding had resulted and that the immediate threat of suicide and death had receded. The treatment contract was regarded to have 'worked' in spite of the fact that she had not complied fully with the contractual agreement. Consequently, discharge from hospital was arranged. At this point Ms Banks broke a mirror in the Unit and used the shards to repeatedly cut her forearms. Feeling frustrated and defeated, the staff felt compelled to shelve the discharge plans.

Treatment contracts require monitoring and if specified goals are not achieved these need discarding, re-negotiating or else discussion to establish why. If the contractual conditions pertaining to the personality disordered patient require them to give up the only defences they have against intolerable feelings, and if no viable alternative outlet or coping strategy is provided or available to them, the contract will not succeed. Therefore it is important that any conditions attached to the contract are realistically achievable. With Ms Banks, it was eventually decided to reinstate and update the treatment contract and to reiterate the need for her to speak in her individual sessions in order to address the maladaptive self-harming behaviour. With regard to the latter, nursing staff's time was made available to her whenever she recognised the impulse to self-mutilate, regardless of the time of day or night.

PRESCRIBING MEDICATION

While psychological treatments of the personality disorder itself form the mainstay, there is a limited role for drug treatment (see Stein, 1992 for review). Symptom disorder and personality disorder comorbidity is common (Du Fort *et al.*, 1993), therefore a substantial proportion of personality disordered patients have a coexisting symptom disorder which may require treatment in its own right, including relevant pharmacotherapy.

In out-patients where impulse control problems are predominant or in-patients who are acutely disturbed or dangerous, there will be a place for the combination of psychotherapy (at least supportive psychotherapy) and pharmacotherapy. However, with many personality disordered patients there is a risk of addiction or of fatal overdose. Under such circumstances there is clearly a need for judicious prescribing. Small doses of an oral neuroleptic, prescribed and dispensed in non-lethal amounts, may represent the safest of medication.

PSYCHOLOGICAL TREATMENTS

If personality disordered patients receive any treatment, it is most likely to be individual supportive psychotherapy (Winston et al., 1994; Monsen et al., 1995). This is not necessarily easy to provide, on an out-patient or in-patient basis, and may require senior and skilled personnel to provide it effectively (see Hartland, 1991). Often, more specialised psychotherapeutic techniques, for example, dynamic psychotherapy, cognitive therapy or dialectical behaviour therapy (Shearer and Linehan, 1994) are required to avoid deterioration in clinical status or to promote beneficial change.

Dynamic psychotherapy aims to facilitate the development of the immature and unintegrated personality through the establishment of a trans-ference–countertransference relationship and its resolution via interpretation as part of a modified, more active, psychoanalytic technique (Kernberg, 1984). Cognitive psychotherapy focuses on the identification of the patient's important cognitive distortions or schemas and examines the way in which these are reiterated and maintained in everyday life. Discussion of such self-defeating and maladaptive manoeuvres is aimed at atrophying their use and replacing them with more self-affirming and adaptive cognitive strategies linked with appropriate affect (for example Young, 1990).

A review of treatment outcome and related issues is beyond the scope of this paper and is available elsewhere (Higgitt and Fonagy, 1992; Stein, 1992; Dolan and Coid, 1993; Norton and Dolan, 1995c; Ruegg and Frances, 1995).

NON-INDIVIDUAL THERAPIES

For a disorder which is known to have such prominent environmental aetiological factors, it is surprising that family therapy is under-represented in the personality disorder literature and perhaps under-utilised as a therapy in clinical practice. This may reflect the absence of an intact family and/or the presence of acrimonious or ambivalent relationships with those family members with whom the patient is still in contact. Sometimes, however, it is not entertained as a treatment because the psychiatrist feels unskilled and/or it is not otherwise available. Family therapy, where family members and treatment resources permit, may have a therapeutic contribution to make, especially in patients' families, which are separation-sensitive or enmeshed.

Box 4 Managing the destructive effect of inter-staff 'splits'

(1) Education of staff regarding the phenomenon of 'splitting' and its inevitable presence in treatment involving more than one staff member and/or agency.

(2) The use of treatment contracts which specify what staff are able and prepared to provide and/or tolerate.

(3) Regular meetings of all relevant staff to identify and resolve differing attitudes to treatment which affect the consistency and speed of its delivery.

(4) Staff support systems for those involved in significant face-to-face contact with PD patients in residential settings.

Reports of the use of group therapy are also under-represented in the literature (Dolan and Coid, 1993), given many personality disordered patients find their way into psychotherapy and clinical psychology departments where they are treated by group dynamic psychotherapeutic methods. The beneficial effect of peer group influences in challenging and shaping personality disordered patients' aberrant or maladaptive attitudes and behaviour, however, is well-established (Bion, 1961; Foulkes, 1964; Tschuschke and Dies, 1994).

SPECIALIST IN-PATIENT UNITS

Referral to a specialist in-patient unit may be indicated where there is: a history of failed outpatient and general psychiatric in-patient treatment; an accumulating number of failed relationships; a poor occupational record and evidence that hopelessness and destructive living styles have become incorporated into the patient's personality (Greben, 1983). Basic educational achievement, a period of stable employment, maintenance of interpersonal stability in an intimate relationship for longer than six months and a recall of a positive enduring relationship during childhood may be good prognostic indicators of a successful outcome with specialist treatment (Whiteley, 1970; Healy and Kennedy, 1993). Any referral and/or transfer, however, needs to be carefully discussed with the personality disordered patient if it is not to be experienced by them as a rejection or as a confirmation of their inherent badness, paradoxically, as confirmation of their untreatability.

One of the advantages of the specialist in-patient unit lies in its power to select its patients and to deploy a coherent and coordinated treatment strategy via staff who have become expert in the particular method. The usual therapeutic emphasis is psychodynamic and in some units no psychotropic medication is prescribed (Norton, 1992). Units vary in the extent to which they utilise the therapeutic influence of the personality disordered patient's peer group (Hinshelwood, 1988; Norton and Dolan, 1995; Reiss et al., 1996). Most require motivated and voluntary participation in treatment and some capacity to experience subjective distress. Treatment lasts between 6 and 18 months and there is accumulating evidence of the success of such units in terms of change in behaviour (Copas et al., 1986; Cullen, 1994) psychological improvement (Dolan et al., 1992; Stone, 1993) and cost-offset following treatment (Dolan et al., 1996).

In spite of such intensive and expert treatment, after-care is often required in many cases of severe personality disorder and treatment may need to be long-term, lasting for a number of years. Information regarding this can be shared with the patient to facilitate engagement in treatment, not least because of its introduction of a realistic time-frame in which treatment goals can be negotiated and tackled. Failure to introduce this aspect early on can contribute to unrealistic expectations and treatment failure, however, such information needs to be imparted sensitively so as not to extinguish all hope or optimism that the patient has in the treatment.

CONCLUSIONS

Many of the clinical needs of personality disordered patients do not differ fundamentally from those of other non-psychotic patients. However, the experience of most psychiatrists is that some of these patients are numbered among the most problematic clinical management problems that they encounter. Characteristically, difficulties arise because the patient is relatively or absolutely unable to perform the role of patient and because clinical issues are supplanted by interpersonal problems. Knowing this can save the psychiatrist some disappointment and frustration since it can lead to education of the patient about the expected role of patients thus keeping expectations of help and treatment within reasonable bounds. This therapeutic endeavour can be helped by the careful and judicious introduction of a treatment contract. The latter serves to bolster the legitimate professional activity by describing the actual limits of the professional input, including the proscription of some of the interpersonal aspects whose distracting presence only undermines the professional level activity. However, there are many pitfalls in the use of treatment contracts which need to be avoided. In the management of any case where there is more than one professional or more than one agency involved, there is a potential for unhelpful 'splitting'. The most regular destructive effect of this is the production of an inconsistent delivery of treatment, regardless of type or model. To avoid this, all relevant staff must meet regularly and, if necessary, frequently, to iron out disagreements or other inconsistencies. Only in this way can the patient experience treatment which is simultaneously emotionally containing and appropriately confronting and challenging.

The marshalling of professional resources, and in some cases those of other patients (as in group, milieu or therapeutic community treatment) or members of the personality disordered patient's wider social network (as in marital and family work), need to be carefully coordinated. Only if this is so can the predictable (external) organisational structure be assimilated by the patient for later internalisation. Well organised and coordinated treatment plans can convey a predictable and responsive experience of the world to patients for whom this was previously lacking. Maintaining such a concerted stance, however, may require specialised in-patient psychotherapeutic management as part of a long-term treatment plan.

ACKNOWLEDGEMENT

I thank Dr Bridget Dolan for her helpful editorial comments and suggested improvements to an earlier draft of this paper.

REFERENCES

Bion, W.R. (1961). *Experience in Groups*. London: Tavistock.

Bowlby, J. (1973). *Attachment and Loss, Vol. 2. Separation: Anxiety and Anger*. New York: Basic Books.

Coid, J.W. (1989). Psychopathic disorders. *Current Opinion in Psychiatry*, 1, p.750–756.

Copas, J.B., O'Brien, M., Roberts, J.C., *et al.* (1986). Treatment outcome in personality disorder: the effect of social, psychological and behavioural variables. *Personality and Individual Differences*, 5, p.565–573.

Cullen, E. (1994). Grendon: the therapeutic prison that works. *Therapeutic Communities*, 15, p.301–311.

Dolan, B., Evans, C. and Wilson, J. (1992). Therapeutic community treatment for personality disordered adults: changes in neurotic symptomatology on follow-up. *International Journal of Social Psychiatry*, 38, p.242–250.

Dolan, B. and Coid, J. (1993). *Psychopathic and Antisocial Personality Disorders: Treatment and Research Issues*. London: Gaskell.

Dolan, B., Evans, C. and Norton, K. (1995). Multiple Axis II diagnosis of personality disorder. *British Journal of Psychiatry*, 166, p.107–112.

Dolan, B., Warren, F., Menzies, D., *et al.* (1996). Cost-offset following specialist treatment of severe personality disorders. *Psychiatric Bulletin*, 20, p.413–417.

Du Fort, C.G., Newman, S.C. and Bland, R.C. (1993). Psychiatric comorbidity and treatment seeking: sources of selection bias in the study of clinical populations. *Journal of Nervous and Mental Diseases*, 18, p.467–474.

Foulkes, S. (1964). *Therapeutic Group Analysis.* London: George Allen & Unwin.

Frank, A.F. (1991). 'The therapeutic alliances of borderline patients.' In J. Clarkin, E. Marziali and H. Munroe-Blum, eds. *Borderline Personality Disorder: Clinical and Empirical Perspectives.* New York: Guilford, p.220–247.

Greben, S. (1983). The multi-dimensional inpatient treatment of severe character disorders. *Canadian Journal of Psychiatry*, 28, p.97–101.

Hartland, S. (1991). 'Supportive psychotherapy.' In J. Holmes, ed. *Textbook of Psychotherapy in Psychiatric Practice.* London: Churchill Livingstone, p.213–235.

Healey, K. and Kennedy, R. (1993). Which families benefit from in-patient psychotherapeutic work at the Cassel Hospital? *British Journal of Psychotherapy*, 9, p.394–404.

Higgitt, A. and Fonagy, P. (1992). Psychotherapy in borderline and narcissistic personality disorder. *British Journal of Psychiatry*, 161, p.23–43.

Hinshelwood, R. (1988). Psychotherapy in an in-patient setting. *Current Opinion in Psychiatry*, 1, p.304–308.

Horwitz, L. (1974). *Clinical Prediction in Psychotherapy.* New York: Jason Aronson.

Kernberg, O.F. (1984). *Severe Personality Disorders: Psychotherapeutic Strategies.* New Haven and London: Yale University Press.

Lockwood, G. (1992). Psychoanalysis and the cognitive therapy of personality disorders. *Journal of Cognitive Psychotherapy*, 6, p.25–42.

Main, T. (1957). The Ailment. *British Journal of Medical Psychology*, 30, p.129–145. Reprinted in T. Main, (1989). *The Ailment and other Psycho-Analytic Essays.* London: Free Association Books.

Masterson, J.F. (1972). *Treatment of the Borderline Adolescent: A Developmental Approach.* New York: Wiley.

Miller, L.J. (1989). Inpatient management of borderline personality disorder: a review and update. *Journal of Personality Disorders*, 3, p.122–134.

Monsen, J.T., Odland, T., Faugh, A., *et al.* (1995). Personality disorders: changes and stability after intensive psychotherapy focusing on affect consciousness. *Psychotherapy Research*, 5, p.33–48.

Norton, K.R.W. (1992). Personality disordered individuals: the Henderson Hospital model of treatment. *Criminal Behaviour and Mental Health*, 2, p.80–191.

Norton, K.R.W. and Smith, S. (1994). *Problems with Patients: Managing Complicated Clinical Transactions.* Cambridge: Cambridge University Press.

Norton, K.R.W. and Dolan, B. (1995a). Acting out and the institutional response. *Journal of Forensic Psychiatry*, 6, p.317–332.

Norton, K.R.W. and Dolan, B. (1995b). 'Personality disorders and parenting.' In M. Gopfert, J. Webster and M. Seeman, eds. *Parental Psychiatric Disorders.* Cambridge: Cambridge University Press, p.219–232.

Norton, K.R.W. and Dolan, B. (1995c). Personality disorder: assessing change. *Current Opinions in Psychiatry*, 8, p.371–375.

Reiss, D., Grubin, D. and Meux, C. (1996). Young 'psychopaths' in special hospitals: treatment and outcome. *British Journal of Psychiatry*, 168, p.99–104.

Reugg, R. and Frances, A. (1995). New research in personality disorders. *Journal of Personality Disorders*, 9, p.1–48.

Shearer, E.N. and Linehan, M. (1994). Dialectical behaviour therapy for borderline personality disorder: theoretical and empirical foundations. *Acta Psychiatrica Scandinavica*, 89 (suppl. 379), p.61–68.

Stanton, A.H. and Schwartz, M.S. (1954). *The Mental Hospital*. New York: Basic Books.

Stein, G. (1992). Drug treatment of the personality disorders. *British Journal of Psychiatry*, 161, p.167–184.

Stone, M.H. (1993). Long-term outcome in personality disorder. *British Journal of Psychiatry*, 162, p.299–313.

Tschuschke, V. and Dies, R.R. (1994). Intensive analysis of therapeutic factors and outcome in long-term in-patient groups. *International Journal of Group Psychotherapy*, 44, p.185–208.

Tyrer, P. (1988). *Personality Disorder, Diagnosis, Management and Care*. London: Wright.

Whiteley, S. (1970). The response of psychopaths to a therapeutic community. *British Journal of Psychiatry*, 166, p.517–529.

Winston, A., Laikin.M., Pollace, J., *et al.* (1994). Short-term psychotherapy of personality disorders. *American Journal of Psychiatry*, 151, p.190–194.

World Health Organization. (1992). *The Tenth Revision of the International Classification of Mental and Behavioural Disorders* (ICD-10). Geneva: WHO.

Yeomans, F. (1993). When a therapist over-indulges a demanding borderline patient. *Hospital and Community Psychiatry*, 44, p.334–336.

Young, J. (1990). *Cognitive Therapy for Personality Disorders: A Schema Focused Approach*. Sarasota, FL: Professional Resources Exchange.

Zimmerman, M. and Coryell, W.H. (1990). Diagnosing personality disorder in the community. *Archives of General Psychiatry*, 47, p.527–531.

Zimmerman, M., Pfohl, B. and Coryell, W.H. (1991). Major depression and personality disorder. *Journal of Affective Disorders*, 22, p.199–210.

13

Problems in the Management of Borderline Patients[*]

Marcus Evans
1998

. . . .

Editors' reflections

The clinical scenarios in the following paper will probably be uncomfortably familiar to readers working in a variety of secure settings. Individuals with personality disorder frequently adopt the psychic defence of projective identification: defending their fragile sense of self by projecting intolerable states of mind externally. The staff's ability to maintain a containing environment, when under the 'fire' of these projections, is essential to avoid them being pressured into acting rather than thinking. Tolerating anxiety and uncertainty can be challenging for staff groups. As a result, staff and the institution may become seduced into adopting group beliefs (over-valued ideas) which shield them from the anxieties induced by this patient group. Unfortunately these over-valued ideas can prevent reflection, and instead a staff 'group response' occurs, which leads to repeated cycles of behaviour between staff, patients and the institution. The 'danger' of this non-thinking action is that important issues, such as risk, can become overlooked as all subscribe instead to the group 'delusion'.

. . . .

[*] Originally published in *Psychoanalytic Psychotherapy, 12*, 1, 17–29. Reprinted here by permission of Taylor and Francis.

Abstract

In this paper some difficulties in the management of borderline patients being treated on two specialist inpatient units will be explored in the light of changes in the health-care system. On these units, nursing staff developed beliefs about care, based on previous experience of difficulties in the clinical area. In many ways, these assumptions about the patient group were based on common-sense. However, when prescribed indiscriminantly, they became 'over-valued' ideas, which acted as a defence against the patients' communications. Nurses stopped thinking about the meaning of the patients' behaviour, and based their actions and behaviour on pre-selected understanding connected with their own defensive needs. The process of introjection and projection necessary for containment was short-circuited, and nurses acted as if they knew what the patients' behaviour meant, rather than wait for meaning to emerge. Despite the patients' denial of their pathology, when they feel their carers have lost touch with the level of their psychological difficulties, they act out in ways which force the nursing-team into action. When the nursing-team reacts without thinking about the meaning of the patients' behaviour, a mindless and often destructive cycle of action and reaction takes place between staff and patients. This cycle goes against the philosophy of both units, which is to help patients to verbalise rather than act-out their difficulties.

INTRODUCTION

A patient is usually admitted to a hospital or psychiatric unit when there is a breakdown in either the patient's psychic equilibrium or the psychic equilibrium of those around him. In addition to the task of caring for the patient physically, the hospital, and in particular the nursing staff, must act as a container for the fragmented and disturbed aspects of the patient's mind. This process is problematic with borderline patients, because of the nature of their internal world and the level of disturbance they require their carers to contain. To relieve the internal turmoil, they use primitive methods of evacuation-communication, in which parts of the patient's internal world is split-off in phantasy and projected into members of the staff-team where it is then believed to be located. However, this is an unstable solution, as projected parts of the patient are always threatening violently to re-enter the patient's internal world, with catastrophic consequences. This leads to dramatic fluctuations in the patient's mental state as he oscillates between a confusing mixture of identities ranging from apparently healthy to disturbed.

The nurse may take the brunt of the patient's anxiety, pain, chaos and madness, in a fairly undiluted way, during acute illnesses, and often for long periods. The nurse's capacity to contain the patient is to some extent affected by institutional beliefs and attitudes about the work. Menzies-Lyth (1959) has described how nursing staff were expected to accept projections of the patient's anxiety, depression, and disgust about his illness. She emphasises the nurse's contact with disease and death, and describes how the objective external situation provides an opportunity for nurses to work through their own internal infantile anxieties. This is possible, provided the external situation is used symbolically, and does not become confused with internal reality.

In her study of student nurses in a general teaching hospital, Menzies-Lyth emphasised the importance of reality-testing in which the difference between internal psychic reality and external reality are continually being worked through, via the patient's contact with the nurse. In contrast to this model, the hospital described in her study developed a social system which aimed to split up the nurses' relationship to their patients in an attempt to protect them from anxiety and pain associated with the work. A rigid social structure developed which prevented nurses from reality-testing and working through their anxieties in relation to their patients, partly because such working-through is so difficult and painful.

On a similar theme, Fabricius (1991) outlined three things which she felt influenced the nurse's capacity to hold the patient:

—the overwhelming quantity and quality of projections,

—the lack of containing structure for the nurse,

—the nurse's own devaluation of her maternal function.

Fabricius coined the term 'running on the spot' to describe a process in which nursing seems endlessly to change its structures in order to defend against anxiety which is inherent in the work.

This paper will start by outlining some general changes in the culture and beliefs of the health-care system. It will then go on to describe two clinical examples taken from specialist units for the treatment of borderline patients in which there has been a breakdown in the relationship between patients and staff. The connection between the breakdown in containment provided, and the staff-teams' defensive assumptions will be explored.

CHANGES IN CULTURE AND BELIEFS IN HEALTH-CARE

Goffman (1961) presented a bleak picture of the institution as a place where patients are stripped of their individuality. He used the term 'institutionalisation' to describe certain regressive tendencies, which he argued were created by institutions. The influence of this study was far reaching, as it indicated that the way people are treated in institutions has a large influence on the way they behave. Perhaps this study, in addition to advances in medical knowledge, has led to a recent shift from an illness model to a health model, in which illness and dependency are presumed to be stigmatising concepts which undermine the individual.

This change in philosophy has been reflected in the enormous shift from institutional to community care over the past fifteen years, and a dramatic reduction in the number of in-patient beds available. Recently, the introduction of the internal market, and extra-contractual referrals for specialist services, has meant that patients and their referrers are seen as the 'paying customer', and as such are entitled to an increasing amount of influence in the way services operate. This change is amplified by the Patients Charter, which outlines patients' rights, and has led to a rise in the number of complaints about psychiatric services.

BORDERLINE PATIENTS IN HOSPITAL

Patients with a diagnosis of borderline personality disorder are often extremely disturbed, and cause severe management problems for psychiatric services, general practitioners, and others. They have little capacity to tolerate frustration, or think symbolically about their emotional life; and they use action to discharge psychic tension. They rely upon primitive forms of projective identification to evacuate unwanted or turbulent parts of their internal world, which involves splitting and projecting parts of the ego. Consequently, their perception of themselves and others is distorted, and leads to difficulties in differentiating between self and other. This in turn means their psychological equilibrium is upset by changes in their environment or separation from the object who contains the split-off part of their ego. These problems are reflected in their relationships which are often chaotic and turbulent.

Characteristically, they may harm themselves in various ways, and many abuse drugs or alcohol, and have little sense of themselves or what they feel. They seek excitement as a way of feeling alive, and are often demanding of service resources, as their self-destructive and chaotic behaviour raises anxiety amongst health-care professionals. It is common for these patients to have large numbers of health-care professionals involved at the same time, and many present themselves as victims of varying kinds of abuse. These accusations help to enlist professionals' sympathy, and stimulate a wish to rescue them. They seek intense, special relationships in which they believe their dependency-needs can be met, and they often push staff beyond the bounds of normal professional behaviour in an attempt to meet these needs.

In hospital, the alarming and dangerous behaviour of patients forces their carers into action which is aimed at protecting them from themselves. Individual members of staff, and at times whole units, are pushed into a situation in which they feel entirely responsible for a patient's actions. For example, the staff may decide to put a patient under close nursing observation. At times this may be appropriate. But it can become a malignant cycle, as the patient projects all responsibility for his wellbeing into the staff. Any attempts to reduce the level of supervision leads to acting-out which in turn puts pressure on staff to increase observations, and may push the team into sectioning the patient. Over time, this situation begins to break down, as staff become increasingly disillusioned and frustrated with the patient for not improving. The staff may feel misled and controlled by the patient, who has raised their expectations, before tormenting them by his failure to improve or develop. Commonly this can become a sado-masochistic relationship in which the patient sadistically attacks the staff's feeling of hope or responsibility by harming himself. The staff may then act-out the sado-masochistic pattern, as their treatment of the patient becomes dominated either by the wish to retaliate or by a guilty compliance with the patient's wishes.

When the team is dominated by a wish for retaliation they sometimes resort to desperate action, often discharging the patient while accusing him of being manipulative and hysterical. His self-destructive behaviour is not taken seriously, and he comes to be looked upon as a naughty child needing to be punished. They decide that the patient is not psychiatrically ill, and agree that he should not have been admitted in the first place. This in turn may lead the patient to behave in dramatic self-destructive ways in an attempt to force staff to continue caring for him; or to complain that the staff have behaved in an abusive and destructive way.

Alternatively, when the team is dominated by masochistic guilt, the patient is given special allowances and is kept in hospital without a clear treatment plan. The staff-team is then left feeling demoralised and trapped by the patient's pathology. They give up any idea of treatment, and resign themselves grudgingly to long-term care of an intransigent patient. Such a patient is often placed in a private hospital on a long-term basis, where he is treated like a paying guest at a hotel, at great expense to the health authority. Alternatively, and relatively rarely, the patient may be referred to a psychiatric unit which specialises in his type of problem.

Working with staff working with borderline patients

I am now going to present two clinical examples taken from weekly work discussion groups I run in different specialist units. Both groups were requested by senior members of the nursing-team and are primarily attended by the nursing-team. The group's task is to think about the nurses' relationships with their patients.

First clinical example

The unit described treated patients who had a history of severe deliberate self-harm and were usually referred to it as a last resort.

A primary nurse presented an incident that had occurred the previous week. Ms A had come to the ward under Section on account of her unmanageable self-destructive behaviour. She presented herself as the victim of various abusive relationships, including her previous psychiatric ward-staff who she accused of maltreating her. The patient's care on the unit was divided between the primary nurse, who concerned herself with the patient's deliberate self-harming behaviour, and an associate nurse who offered 'abuse counselling'. This seemed to be a supportive relationship, in which the patient was seen to be the innocent victim of neglect or abuse. The associate nurse reported that the patient's stay had been going well, until this point. She emphasised that Ms A was an extremely capable and likable woman who showed tremendous potential as an artist. The primary nurse was more reticent about Ms A's progress, and mentioned that the deliberate self-harming behaviour had continued on a regular and increasingly frequent basis. As a consequence of her 'progress' on the ward, Ms A had been taken off her Section as part of her preparation for discharge.

Ms A then discussed a shopping trip with her primary nurse, giving assurance that she would not visit her ex-boyfriend who was known to be violent. Ms A left the ward and was brought back by the Police the next day, having been severely assaulted by her boyfriend. The primary nurse described how she had to sit in with the patient while the doctor examined Ms A's beaten body. As she told the group about her experiences, she was visibly shaken, and finished by saying she was disgusted by the damage done, and did not know if she was cut out for this type of work.

In discussion, several problems about Ms A's management emerged. Her self-destructive behaviour had encouraged previous institutions to take responsibility for keeping her alive by putting her on continuing close observations under Section. This became an unhelpful malignant pattern as Ms A became increasingly dependent upon institutions to care for her. When she was admitted to the unit they hoped to reverse the trend by encouraging her to act in a more adult and responsible way. This was reflected in their decision to remove her Section Order. Ms A gave the impression of being intelligent, artic-ulate, and motivated to cooperate with the plan. However, her improvement seemed to be based on a rather fragile pseudo-adult facade which kept the ward staff at some distance from her pathology. The abuse counsellor seemed to go along with a split that existed in the patient, in which all pathology was projected by the patient into past or external figures who she felt had failed her. This split was mirrored in the staff's relationships with the patient, as her actions and self-harming behaviour were dealt with by one nurse, while responsibility for abuse counselling was dealt with by another. Thus, the patient's re-enactment of sado-masochistic and abusive relationships in the transference with the ward were split-off from the abuse counselling, as if the two were unrelated.

The patient's apparent improvement was sustainable as long as the ward continued to care for Ms A. The moment they decided to remove the Section Order and to plan her discharge, Ms A's pseudo-adult facade collapsed as she reverted to her previous sado-masochistic state of mind. As well as punishing the ward, Ms A's actions can be seen as an attempt to show staff that she needed to feel they understood the level of her difficulties.

In previous work discussions, I had been alarmed by the staff's apparent lack of anxiety in relation to the high incidence and seriousness of patients' self-harming behaviour. I frequently became concerned that patients were forced to escalate their self-harming behaviour in an attempt to get the nursing-staff to take things seriously. The patients on the unit had very little capacity to tolerate frustration or metabolise and articulate their psychological state; and they used action to evacuate undigested psychological experience. In the example above, different parts of the patient were communicated to different parts of the nursing-team.

The nursing staff's capacity to think about, and make sense of, their patients is a dynamic process relying upon numerous factors, including the team's capacity to verbalise and integrate the views of the patient. This is a potentially turbulent process, requiring a constant examination of the nurse's contact with the patient, within an atmosphere of curiosity and openness. It also means that the staff-team have to tolerate doubt and uncertainty about their work, while the process goes on. When treating such disturbed patients, doubt and anxiety are difficult to bear, and teams often search for explanations which provide structure and certainty.

Bion (1967) thought psychic change was connected with the discovery of a selected fact. The selected fact is a linking observation making sense of facts which were previously seen as disparate: in other words, a new and previously unseen pattern emerging from the patient's material surrounding a particular clinical fact. Bion described the circumstances in which a selected fact emerges. The therapist waits in a state of expectation, with all his theories and previous experiences, and these are the therapist's preconceptions. The therapist then takes in communications until he finds a sense-impression of the patient which fits with a preconception. Once this happens, a selected fact is born.

Britton and Steiner (1994) have continued this theme by describing some of Bion's ideas about the relationship between the selected fact and what they describe as the 'over-valued idea'. The 'over-valued idea', or pre-selected fact, is a cluster of apparently related facts surrounding a hypothesis in the therapist's mind, which masquerade as a new and genuine development in understanding. In the case of the over-valued idea, the integration is spurious, and results from the facts being forced together into a hypothesis or theory which the therapist needs for defensive purposes. For example, the over-valued idea can be used by the therapist to give a sense of integration to otherwise disparate and confusing experiences. Britton and Steiner describe two reasons for the emergence of an over-valued idea in preference to waiting in uncertainty for a 'selected fact' to emerge:

Firstly, the patient is disturbed by uncertainties, and puts pressure on the therapist to find meaning in his experience. The patient may also be extremely sensitive to the therapist's way of thinking, and may present material or interpret the therapist's behaviour in conformity with certain unconscious beliefs he has about himself, thus constricting the therapy; and, secondly, in a situation of uncertainty and confusion the therapist relieves his fear of losing his identity by attaching himself to an over-valued idea for which he seeks con-firmation in the patient. These beliefs are often unconsciously necessary for the therapist.

In the unit described above, the nurses' thinking seemed to be based on a belief that Ms A's behaviour was caused by low self-esteem and insecurity, caused by previous abusive relationships. The unit tried to provide a non-abusive situation in which the patient could build her self-esteem and con-sequently relinquish the help-seeking, destructive, self-harming behaviour. The unit saw the patient as a victim of abuse who needed to disentangle herself from previous abusive relationships, thus encouraging a split between a healthy part of the patient that was the victim of abuse and consequently low self-esteem, and a destructive part of the patient identified with an abuser in the patient's past. This split denied the patient's involvement in abusive and perverse states of mind, and also ignored the re-enactment of abusive relationships in the transference relationships to the staff. The patient's acting-out was largely ignored in an attempt to avoid malignant cycles of care established by previous institutions. Emphasis instead was put on the intense individual relationship with the patient and her verbal communication. All communication and pathology contained in the acting-out was ignored at the expense of the patient's verbal communications.

In order to prevent the malignant patterns of care established by these patients in previous units, staff developed a hardened attitude towards their patients and refused to be dominated by their behaviour. They projected all anxiety about their approach into staff in other parts of the hospital, who were seen as either weak and unskilled in their management of these patients, or judgemental and disapproving of the unit's philosophy. This siege mentality inhibited the ward's own thinking and capacity critically to evaluate their approach.

In his study of groups, Bion (1962) outlined his belief that all groups oscillate between two contrasting states of mind. The work-group mentality describes a situation in which the group applies itself thoughtfully to the agreed task and involves the group learning from experience through testing its thinking against reality. In contrast, the basic-assumption group mentality is a state of mind which opposes the group task and involves omnipotent ways of thinking, and which requires no training, or capacity to learn from experience.

Now it seems a legitimate aim of psychiatric services dealing with regressive and dysfunctional behaviour to encourage patients to take responsibility for their actions. But current assumptions about the stigma of illness and dependence may be acting in ways which defend staff and services from the full impact of their problem by encouraging a 'supermarket mentality', in which providers are encouraged aggressively to market their produce in order to win orders. This can encourage providers to make claims for their treatments which are unrealistic, given the patients' psychopathology; and this inevitably leads to disappointment and demoralisation of the service.

Second clinical example

I was asked to run a work-discussion group for an in-patient unit which functioned as a medium- to long-stay facility for patients with a personality disorder, most of whom had been under the care of the hospital for some time. The unit was scheduled for closure within six months, despite the fact that it had a high profile in its specialty and a reputation for taking the most difficult patients. As a specialty, the unit could not guarantee its survival in the internal market as it had high running costs related to the length of patients' stay and the high level of supervision required by this patient group. The unit also saw itself as being psychoanalytically enlightened.

Soon after starting the group, I became disturbed by the nature of the relationship between staff and patients on the unit. Each patient had his own key nurse who was responsible for coordinating his care. These relationships were highly valued by staff and patients alike. Indeed, there was considerable competition between patients for attention from different staff-members. Generally, the staff seemed to be over-involved with, and tyrannised by, the patients; indeed, the high incidence of self-harming behaviour led to an atmosphere of malice. I was struck by the level of violence and threatening behaviour displayed by patients towards staff; and on several occasions patients attacked staff verbally and physically.

These outbursts were generally met by appeasement and reinforcement of the idealised relationship. This attitude was reflected in the wider institution, where certain patients seemed to have a celebrity status. There seemed little or no evidence of the staff's capacity to think about their relationships with patients; and staff seemed to act in a boundary-less way, constantly at the beck-and-call of their patients. On one occasion, a weary staff-member came in on his day off to escort a patient on an outing, his reasons for coming in being readily accepted by the staff-group without question.

Two months before the ward was due to close, a bomb was found on the ward amongst the patients' property. After some time, I commented on the relationship between the bomb, various violent acts which had taken place on the ward that week, and the patients' feelings of anger towards the staff related to the wards' closure. Characteristically, my comment was largely but politely ignored. Next week I became even more alarmed to discover that the incident had been almost completely forgotten. When I asked what had happened about the bomb, I was told that the hospital administrators had probably forgotten to inform the Police. When I remarked on the group's lack of concern, I was again largely ignored and left feeling guilty for trying to frighten them by making such a fuss.

Many of the patients saw the unit as a sanctuary for life, and any idea of their moving on provoked acting-out that sabotaged the threat of development. Indeed, one notorious patient had been on special observations for almost two years continuously and threatened to harm herself whenever the observations were reduced. At times in the group, I felt outraged by the mistreatment of patients and tyranny of the staff, and frustrated by the staff's masochistic behaviour.

What emerged during the course of the group was an unspoken, but deeply influential, set of assumptions that the group of patients had been maternally deprived and could be cured by unconditional love. The unit team saw itself as providing a caring environment in which the missing maternal components could be replaced. Now this is a well-researched and respectable explanation for psychological disturbance; but on the unit it had become an 'over-valued' idea, which precluded the emergence of new facts or explanations for patients' behaviour. Acts of violence by patients towards themselves or others were seen as understandable in terms of the assumption that the patients were basically deprived, and craved love and attention. This seemed to provide a way of normalising the patients' behaviour and making the staff's contact with patients more bearable, an idea which the patients were more than happy to promote. It also went along with the patients' infantile wish for an ideal object that would not leave them until previous damage and deprivation had been put right.

There was no room in the staff's idealised view of themselves to accept the limitations of their service, or the limitations of the hospital's resources. The group often discussed their anger with the hospital administration for closing the ward without questioning them or the value of their approach. The acceptance of their patients' behaviour seemed connected to the staff's identifications with the patients' infantile feeling of entitlement and rage towards the hospital for closing the ward. This compliant attitude seemed to encourage patients to act as if the unit and hospital were guilty of negligence or abuse, and consequently deserved punishment. This attitude encouraged a situation in which the patients' feelings of anger, remorse and sadness related to the lost 'ideal' object could be avoided. Staff and patients all colluded in the belief that the 'ideal' object should always be available, and the patients' rage towards the failed 'ideal' object was justified. This was complicated by perverse elements in the patient group which acted to maintain the situation through cruelty towards the staff.

I think I had been asked onto the ward to contain the staff's anxieties that discharging their patients might provoke the most almighty explosion and backlash related to the patients' feeling that they had been misled and betrayed by staff. But knowledge about the full extent of the patients' perverse murderous and destructive wishes, which could not be contained within the idealised relationship, were split-off and projected into me. I was left with the responsibility for worrying about the safety of the patients and staff on the ward; and with the feeling of frustration at the ward's lack of interest in my observations and doubtful about my effectiveness.

In both units, I felt my role was to contain the staff's anxieties about their work, while remaining relatively ineffectual in terms of the wards' general approach or clinical decisions. In some ways, this may represent a repetition of a split in the patients' parental couple, which the patients then recreate in their relationships.

DISCUSSION

Many of the patients in these two units have internal worlds inhabited by cruel, mocking or perverse figures. Rosenfeld (1987) described how the borderline patients' internal world functioned like a well-organised gang which defends the patient from anxieties associated with fragmentation or integration. External relationships are often recruited in ways which support the internal psychic structure. The patient's defensive organisation can remain quite stable until something in the internal or external structure breaks down.

In this state of mind, the patient often feels threatened and overwhelmed by anxiety, and may doubt his capacity to differentiate between inside and outside. Frightened by internal turmoil, the patient seeks a way of regaining control of his internal world by projecting or evacuating parts of the self (in phantasy) into external objects (which then act as a container). Once on the unit, the patient often forms an intense relationship with his primary nurse, who sees herself as offering the support and care the patient needs. In her study Menzies-Lyth (1959) connected the nurse's desire to nurse with her need to repair infantile internal objects damaged by hostility.

Problems arise for nurses when anxieties about their capacity to make repa-ration towards their damaged internal objects becomes confused with the damaged patients in external reality. When this happens, nurses may feel over-whelmed by feelings of despair and helplessness about the impossibility of their task, and feel persecuted by patients who come to represent damaged and reproachful internal objects whom they cannot help. Nurses frequently resort to primitive defences against anxiety based on omnipotent solutions, in order to 'cure' the patients and relieve their own internal anxieties about their capacity for reparation.

Borderline patients present particular problems for nurses in this area, as they hate acknowledging the extent of their pathology that leaves them feeling dependent and humiliated, and they put pressure on staff to provide omnipo-tent solutions to their difficulties. A collusion develops between staff and patients in which healthy aspects of the patients are mobilised to form a fragile adult facade which often fits in with staff's and patients' wishes and expecta-tions. Meanwhile the disturbed and pathological aspect of the patient is split-off and expressed through action. Staff and patients turn a blind eye to the full extent of pathology by paying too much attention to the patients' verbal communication, at the expense of the non-verbal communication.

The primary nurse–patient relationship then takes the form of a pseudo-therapy, in which potentially serious issues are discussed in the absence of any real disturbance, as words become a devalued currency. Patients push the primary nurse into particular patterns of behaviour which may support a fragile adult identification based on an idealised relationship. This is made up of elements of the patient's adult self in identification with the member of staff. Joseph (1985) describes how patients behave in ways which nudge the analyst into behaviour which fits with their expectations and defensive needs. Borderline patients are sensitive also to the defensive needs of their object, and may use this knowledge for further control. This relationship is often driven by the patients' and staff's wish to deny the feelings of pain, anxiety and despair about the level of pathology and disturbance, and the wish for an ideal relationship which will cure the patient of their pathology. It may also be driven by the staff's wish to avoid being accused of abuse or impotence by the patient.

In the two units mentioned, it was my impression that the more disturbed patients had generally improved, while they remained in control of the treatment situation. This was established by a mixture of seduction and threat, similar to the situation described by Main (1957). Certain sympathetic staff were seen as understanding, and were chosen by patients to be their special nurses, and this position left these nurses feeling wanted and important. Pressure was established by a threat that the staff-member would be demoted from her special status if she did not comply with the patient's wishes, and this was always backed up by the threat of acting-out.

The units developed different approaches to a similar patient group, but shared certain characteristics which I shall now outline. Both units believed that the patients had been mistreated by previous carers, and mismanaged by health-care services; and developed a view of the patients as victims of neglect or abuse. They attempted to provide a non-abusive environment which took the patients' grievances seriously and provided appropriate 'therapy' in the belief that they could avoid previous accusations and negative relationships. Indeed, the units saw themselves as being psychotherapeutically enlightened, and there was an idealisation of 'therapeutic' relationships, despite the staff's relative lack of experience, training or supervision.

Both units saw themselves as offering care superior to that of the ordinary psychiatric units, which had 'misunderstood' these patients. This mentality included the projection of their own doubts and anxieties about their approach into the external hospital and an over-estimation of their own capacities which left their thinking impaired. In the first example, this rather superior state of mind seemed to be encouraged by the internal market, which demanded that units sold themselves as offering expertise in order to survive. Developing expertise in this difficult area requires a long-term view of staff-development, and takes many years of expert supervision and training.

The short-term nature of patients' financial contracts encouraged a rather shallow view of the psychopathology of the patients whose difficulties also required a long-term view. In the second example, the staff-team also seemed reluctant to face the full extent of the patients' psychopathology, and there was a compliance with the patients' insistence that they should never be expected to care for themselves unless they had been cured. This refusal to accept the reality of patients' psychopathology and damage is reflected also in the current culture within the health-care system which tends to encourage a 'normalised' view of psychiatric illness, in the belief that the stigma of mental illness is damaging. While this is doubtless true, it is also damaging to underestimate the extent of the patients' psychopathology and need.

CONCLUSION

Borderline patients have difficulties dealing with the psychic contents of their minds, and tend to evacuate undigested elements of their minds through action. They also put considerable pressure on nursing staff to act, rather than think. Ideally, the function of the nursing team with these patients is to use their verbal capacity to reverse the process and turn the action, and pressure towards action, back into words. Both units described in this paper tried to offer 'therapy' in order to break this cycle of action and reaction. But their thinking was limited by certain beliefs.

Containment is a mental task involving the capacity to take in and digest the patients' experience without jumping to premature conclusions. To avoid this painful and difficult process, the units described developed 'over-valued' ideas, which short-circuited the process of communication between patient and nurse. In this state of mind, the nurse acts as if she knows what she is doing—certainty in an otherwise chaotic and frightening world. One casualty of the 'over-valued' idea is curiosity, which requires the tolerance of doubt and the frustration of not knowing. Current assumptions about the stigma of illness and dependence may also be acting in defensive ways which encourage omnipotent solutions within the Health Service as a whole. This group of patients requires a long-term view of their needs, which includes a realistic appreciation of their pathology. They also demand a great deal of their carers, and on-going supervision and training is essential.

REFERENCES

Bion, W.R. (1962). *Experiences in Groups*. London: Tavistock.

Bion, W.R. (1967). *Second Thoughts*. London: Heinemann/Karnac; New York: Aronson.

Britton, R. and Steiner, J. (1994). Interpretation: Selected fact or over-valued idea? *International Journal of Psychoanalysis*, 75, p.1069–1078.

Fabricius, J. (1991). Running on the spot or can nursing really change? *Psychoanalytic Psychotherapy*, 5, p.97–108.

Goffman, E. (1961). *Asylums*. New York: Doubleday; Harmondsworth: Penguin.

Joseph, B. (1985). Transference, the total situation. *International Journal of Psycho-Analysis*, 66, p.447–454. Reprinted in (1989), *Selected Papers of Betty Joseph*. London: Routledge.

Main, T. (1957). The Ailment. *British Journal of Medical Psychology*, 30, p.129–145 and in J. Johns, ed., (1989). *The Ailment and other Psychoanalytic Essays*. London: Free Association Books.

Menzies-Lyth, I. (1959). 'The functioning of social systems as a defence against anxiety.' In (1988), *Containing Anxiety in Institutions*. London: Free Association Books.

Rosenfeld, H. (1987). *Impasse and Interpretation*. London: Tavistock.

ACKNOWLEDGEMENT

I would just like to thank Sue Evans for her help in writing this article.

14

Ten Traps for Therapists in the Treatment of Trauma Survivors[*]

James A. Chu
1988

· ·

Editors' reflections

Whilst this paper is not specifically on the subject of personality disorder, as we have learnt from previous papers in this volume and from clinical experience, the majority (if not all), of our service users will have survived traumatic assaults from others, usually in childhood, and from those they considered 'carers'. Being a therapist for these 'survivors' can be a daunting and confusing mental and emotional experience, and these are feelings which are not just confined to the inexperienced therapist. This paper is extremely useful and accessible; due to Chu's simplicity of writing, and his ability to illustrate 'traps' which occur almost universally when working with service users. We have found Chu's practical approach to these concepts particularly appealing, as it brings the material to life and is easily 'translated' to clinical practice. The uncovering and overcoming of 'traps' is an essential component of therapy and this paper offers rich material that reminds us to constantly 'monitor ourselves' in our therapeutic task. Although individual therapy is the focus here, the 'traps' described are likely to occur in other forms of therapy, and Chu's ideas may well be usefully extended to institutions and organisations.

· ·

[*] Originally published in *Dissociation*, 1, 4, 24–32. Reprinted here by permission of James A. Chu.

Abstract

Patients who have survived trauma, particularly those who have experienced early childhood abuse, stand out in the clinical experience of many therapists as being among the most difficult patients to treat. These patients have particular patterns of relatedness, along with intense neediness and dependency which make them superb testers of the abilities of their therapists. They often push therapists to examine the rationales and limits of their therapeutic abilities, and frequently force therapists to examine their own personal issues and ethical beliefs. A conceptual framework for understanding treatment traps is presented, along with ten traps which these patients present, consciously or unconsciously, in the course of treatment. Included are traps around trust, distance, boundaries, limits, responsibility, control, denial, projection, idealization, and motivation. These are certainly not the only traps which occur in the course of treatment, but they highlight the experience of treatment and the difficulties which are encountered between the therapist and the patient. This paper is intended to be clinical in orientation to help prepare and support therapists in their work.

INTRODUCTION

Trauma survivors, particularly those with histories of early childhood physical and sexual abuse, seem to be among the most distressed patients (Bryer *et al.* 1987) and often the most difficult to treat. They present in a variety of ways with dissociative disorders, borderline states, substance abuse, eating disorders, and various syndromes of anxiety and depression. My own experience in working with such patients and in consulting and supervising their therapists, confirms that difficulties occur frequently, repeatedly, and with remarkable predictability. Other investigators, such as Kluft (1984), have also described therapists experiencing "bewilderment, exasperation, and a sense of being drained" (p.51). This paper describes the nature of certain therapeutic impasses or "traps" in their psychotherapy, and outlines a conceptual framework as to why such traps are particularly difficult with trauma survivors. Ten common clinical traps are also presented along with suggestions for intervention. One caveat: an understanding of the traps does not prevent them from occurring. However, an understanding prevents therapists from becoming enmeshed in traps, and helps therapists tolerate them with less anxiety.

THE NATURE OF TREATMENT TRAPS

In treatment traps, or therapeutic impasses, often both the patient and therapist feel immobilized. In these difficult clinical situations the therapy is brought to a standstill or even regresses. These kinds of treatment traps seem to arise from resistances brought by patients to the therapy. However, in that psychotherapy involves interaction in an interpersonal arena, traps are fully activated only if the therapist responds inadequately or inappropriately to these resistances. Resistances throughout the course of treatment are normal and expectable. Unless such resistances are acknowledged by both the patient and the therapist, an impasse or unfortunate clinical result occurs (Glover, 1955; Greenson, 1967; Langs, 1981). Appropriate responses on the part of the therapist allows resistances to be understood and resolved. Greenson (1967) defines the steps which are often necessary to resolve resistances as confrontation, clarification, interpretation, and working through. In other words, both patient and therapist need to acknowledge and consider the resistant behaviors, understand them on a conscious level, and to make progressive changes. If this occurs, the therapy is enhanced, but without an appropriate resolution, the therapy flounders.

What leads therapists to make non-therapeutic responses to manifestations of patient resistance? Inexperienced or naive therapists often overlook evidence of resistance. Even experienced therapists, on occasion, can miss or misunderstand evidence of resistance, and can find themselves in difficult clinical straits. Often, however, the difficulty in dealing with patient's resistances are due to more complex therapist dynamics. The therapist's countertransference, that is, the therapist's own thoughts, feelings, and wishes which are projected into the patient, may interfere with productive interventions. Langs (1981) has stated that: "it is incumbent upon the therapist to ascertain his own contributions to each resistance before dealing with those sources which arise primarily from the patient" (p.540). Not understanding countertransference contributions in relation to patient resistance (either in promoting resistance or in response to resistance) almost certainly leads to nontherapeutic responses. Such responses might range from feeling immobilized, to rage at being attacked, to being overgratified by the patient. One other area of therapist contribution to treatment traps comes from therapists' counterresistance (Glover, 1955). Patients in therapy may activate thoughts, feelings and fantasies in their therapists which their therapists attempt to fend off. Thus, therapists' counterresistances, particularly in trying to cope with angry reactions or sadistic fantasies towards patients, can lead to therapists using such defenses as reaction formation, avoidance or withdrawal. Strean (1985) mentions possible forms counter-resistance can take: "oversolicitousness; unnecessary reassurances; ...postponing confrontations, questions or interpretations regarding a client's tardiness or absence; glossing over... the negative transference; and denying the existence of pathology, conflict, or resistance in the client" (p.85).

TRAPS IN THE TREATMENT OF TRAUMA SURVIVORS

The painful difficulties that inevitably appear in the treatment of trauma survivors seem to be the result of two factors, the first having to do with particular characteristics of these patients. Many trauma survivors who later develop psychiatric disorders have come from highly pathological family backgrounds. Many investigators cite trauma victims' social environment and the reactions (or lack of reaction) to abuse as critical in the long term sequelae (Finkelhor, 1984; Herman, 1981; Russell, 1986). Psychopathology within the family as is the case with incestuous abuse, lack of familial support, or unsupportive reactions from the family to the abuse all seem to contribute to long term difficulties. Spiegel (1986) describes the "double bind" of abused children who later develop dissociative disorders. The child receives totally contradictory messages (such as being both "loved" and abused) and is forbidden from addressing the contradictions. The family which nurtures the child is also the source of abuse, abandonment, and betrayal. It is hence not surprising that trauma survivors have enormously impaired abilities to engage in a therapeutic relationship with a therapist to help resolve their difficulties.

As a result of their abusive backgrounds, many trauma survivors have extraordinary manifestations of resistance (Chu, 1988). Many of these patients use extensive repression and dissociation, which may make it difficult for the patient to consciously know, much less communicate, the nature of his or her difficulties. Moreover, these patients are understandably resistant to the necessary work of exploration and retrieval of very painful and intolerable experiences. The powerful resistances of trauma survivors lead them to engage with therapists in particular ways. Many such patients, who are often bright, articulate and creative, can be extremely persuasive in arguing for certain directions in treatment or in the gratification of certain needs. Although often correct in the assessment of their own felt needs, patients may lead therapists to ignore underlying resistances, vulnerabilities, errors in judgement, possible detrimental consequences, or even the therapist's own needs.

The second factor leading to treatment traps with trauma survivors has to do with therapists' contributions. The extreme pain of past experiences and the reservoir of overwhelming affect may, at times, be nearly as difficult for the therapist as for the patient. In addition, many patients have highly fragmented

personality structures and poor ego functioning, resulting in profound dependency and neediness. The need not to be alone, the need to know more about the
therapist in order to feel secure, the need to be loved and cared about, are all too
urgent and genuine. It is normative for therapists to want to deny, distance and
withdraw on the one hand, and to want to gratify need, soothe, comfort and
rescue patients on the other. Such feelings of the therapist, if unrecognized,
make the therapist the unwitting partner in actions which often lack perspective and judgement, to the detriment of the patient, the therapist, and the
treatment. Treatment traps often occur with the combination of the patient's
acute distress, the emerging of overwhelming past traumatic experiences, fierce
resistances as the patient finds the treatment itself painful, and extreme difficulty in maintaining a therapeutic alliance. It is no wonder that therapists have
difficulty in managing their own responses and reactions to patients in crisis,
and repeatedly find themselves conflicted, confused, frustrated, intimidated,
anxious, and frightened. Nonetheless, particularly early in treatment, when the
patient most lacks overall perspective, it falls to the therapist to make informed
decisions about treatment. Although the therapy could not (and should not)
proceed without extensive input from patient, it remains the responsibility of
the therapist to assess the needs of the patient, the wisdom of any particular
course of action, the consequences of such action, the realities of the environment, and the limitations of therapy and the therapist. The discussion and
clinical illustrations below are intended to give some framework to making
such decisions. In all cases, the identity of patients and therapists have been
disguised. Patients are referred to in the feminine gender, as the majority of
these patients who present for treatment appear to be women.

Trap #1: trust

The most common trap for therapists, particularly those unfamiliar with the
treatment of trauma survivors, is the assumption of the presence of trust. It is
crucial to recognize that patients who have backgrounds of abuse, neglect, and
abandonment, often at the hands of their caretakers, do not know the meaning
of trusting human relationships. In fact, the inability to establish and maintain
healthy relationships based on mutuality is a primary disability of many such
patients. Many discussions of treatment in the multiple personality disorder literature (often involving the treatment of patients who have been severely and
extensively abused) make explicit the need for the establishment of trust
(Braun, 1986; Wilbur, 1984). However, a reasonable level of trust often takes
months or years to develop, and a normal level of trust usually exists only when
the treatment nears its end. Throughout the therapy patients repeatedly test

their therapists, and therapists find themselves trying to demonstrate, both verbally and behaviorally, that trust is possible. The problem is particularly painful given that not only does the patient not have any reasonable notion of trust, but fully expects betrayal of trust, and will look for any evidence of untrustworthiness on the part of the therapist. When a crisis inevitably occurs because the patient perceives some reason, reality based or not, to mistrust the therapist, the therapist is required to have the patience to weather the storm rather than to make superhuman efforts to prove trustworthiness, or to withdraw in frustration. On the positive side, patients usually desperately wish to be able to trust, and are aware that others around them are capable of trusting and engaging with people in a way that they are not. However, this may also lead to their presenting a facade of trusting, and the development of trust must always be measured by the patient's actions as well as words.

Case illustration

A young woman was progressing well in therapy over the first six months with her therapist, and had had a marked reduction in self-mutilating activity. This was largely accomplished by weekly contracts with her therapist not to hurt herself. Although she talked with her therapist, she did not allow her most angry and regressed sides to emerge. She was still vague, and perhaps secretive, about details of her background, only hinted about numerous episodes of childhood abuse. However, the patient was symptomatically better, appeared more comfortable at home and at work, and spoke optimistically about her future. Following a therapy session one week, the therapist realized that he had neglected to renew the weekly contract, but decided to take no action feeling that enough trust had been established to make contracting unnecessary. The patient, on the other hand, feeling certain that this oversight was a sign that her therapist was losing interest and soon planned to terminate with her, make a serious suicide attempt, resulting in hospitalization. The therapist became quite frustrated and angry, and talked to the hospital staff about the patient's "attention seeking behavior" and lack of motivation to improve.

Trap #2: distance

In response to patients' resistance to trusting, therapists may respond by becoming distant. Certainly, in the face of overwhelming neediness and constant pleas for reassurance, therapists may understandably feel the urge to withdraw. Therapists who have been trained in the psychoanalytic tradition, where distance and passivity are deliberately used to encourage transference phenomena, may particularly vulnerable to withdrawing. However, it is worth considering whether distance is appropriate for patients who have major problems in maintaining basic relationships. For patients who have been previously abandoned and traumatized, the distance may simply be a recapitulation of their previous experience of being left alone. Mays and Franks (1985), in discussing negative outcomes in who they define as "high risk patients" (many of which share characteristics of trauma survivors), recommend matching such patients with "therapists who are able to sustain the highest levels of empathy, warmth, and genuineness" (p.294). Chessick's (1982) "existential alliance" classification seems most appropriate for patients with traumatic histories, in which the therapist provides a real interpersonal sharing of the patient's experiences. In this sense, the therapist must be a participant as well as an observer in the therapeutic relationship. It is very helpful for therapists to see the therapeutic relationship as a dynamic, interpersonal arena in which both parties participate, rather than seeing only the patient and the patient's behavior as determining the nature of the relationship. In clinical practice, during times of crisis within the relationship, very often what is required is for the therapist to move closer to the patient rather than to become more distant. This often has the effect of reducing or eliminating the crisis in the treatment. However, therapists often find themselves moving further away from what they see as inappropriate neediness and dependency on the part of their patients. This frequently results in harm to the patient, to the therapy, and flight from treatment.

Case illustration

A woman in her forties had been in psychotherapy for the major part of her adult life. It was known she had a sexual abuse history, but this was unacknowledged in most of her therapies. Her current therapy consisted of once a week with a male therapist who worked in a very traditional manner. All attempts on the patient's part to get the therapist more involved in her treatment were met with an increasing sense of distance. The patient was quite chronically angry at her therapist but felt so dependent on him that she largely repressed her anger. Symptomatically she did not improve and continued to have bouts of anxiety, depression and rage, at times engaging in self-destructive behavior. She began to quarrel with the therapist over appointment times and telephone calls during the session. The therapist seemed to respond by becoming more erratic in scheduling appointment times and insisting on taking telephone calls during the session. Finally, towards the end of one meeting, the patient had the overwhelming sensation of being strangled by her father. She felt physically choked and panicked. As she struggled to let the therapist know what she was experiencing, the therapist got out of his chair, turned his back, and announced that the time was up. The patient left therapy shortly after this incident.

Trap #3: boundaries

Children who are abused usually come from families which provide extremely inconsistent nurturing (Spiegel, 1986) and where family roles are grossly distorted (Herman, 1981). Interpersonal boundaries in the therapy are extremely important as the patient has little idea of what to expect from the therapist. For example, in the transference, a patient might expect even a warm and nurturing therapist to turn and strike her, or may constantly be on guard for a role reversal where the therapist looks to the patient for nurturing. It is this lack of trust and this not knowing what to expect that often leads patients to push interpersonal boundaries. The patient may feel strongly that to know more and participate more in the therapist's life will lead to more security and trust, and may attempt to convince or coerce the therapist into revealing personal details. Willingness to provide a certain amount of self-disclosure and reflection of feelings may be extremely helpful to some patients (Richert, 1983). However, boundaries are essential wherever they are placed. Therapists may choose where the boundaries are to be placed, according to his or her style and comfort, but must recognize that they are essential to helping the patient maintain control and perspective. The self-perceived need for reassurance on the part of the patient is endless, and issues around trust will arise no matter where the boundaries are placed. The wise therapist realizes that it is stabilizing in the long run to be clear about boundaries, and for patients to realistically understand the nature of the relationship. Furthermore, therapists need to feel personally comfortable with boundaries that protect their privacy in order to function effectively as therapists.

Case illustration

Over the course of several months a patient pushed her therapist to tell her more about the therapist's personal life so that she could feel more secure in the relationship. Repeatedly, the patient asked the therapist to tell her how the therapist managed her problems so that the patient could have a better grasp on how to manage hers. Over time, the patient became intimately acquainted with the details of the therapist's life, including her marital relationship. Although the therapist was increasingly uncomfortable with these intrusions into her personal life, she allowed them to continue, feeling strongly committed to showing her patient that she cared and could be trusted. She feared saying anything that would make the patient angry, and occasionally was also secretly gratified at the opportunity to talk about some of her own problems. However, when the patient began appearing at the therapist's home, the therapist informed her that she would not permit this, and would no longer discuss any matters pertaining to her personal life. The result was a stormy interchange in which the patient accused the therapist of abusing her by leading her to expect that she could be a part of the therapist's personal life. She questioned the therapist's ability to follow through with any of her promises, as well as the therapist's competence, commitment, and caring. Knowing a great deal about the therapist's personal life, the patient suggested that the therapist's marital relationship was unstable, and that the therapist was using her to gratify unmet needs. The therapist was immobilized with anger, anxiety and confusion.

Trap #4: limits

Closely related to the trap of failing to establish boundaries is the failure to set limits. Part of the treatment of many patients, and particularly traumatized patients with very dysfunctional behaviors, is to provide a containing environment. "Good enough holding" (Winnicott, 1965) often involves appropriate limits to contain dysfunctional behaviors. Although the treatment of these patients requires thoughtful flexibility, there is no need to endlessly gratify patients' demands. Not only does this allow potentially dangerous behaviors, but demonstrates to the patient that even excessive needs can be met, and that no change is necessary to meet the demands of reality. Too often therapists find themselves so identified with the patient's experience that they become immobilized along with the patient. Therapists may also be invested in providing corrective emotional experiences for patients with a history of deprivation, and hence may fear replicating what patients see as depriving or abusive experiences. Even extreme efforts to meet patients' demands and to avoid patients' anger usually fail. All too often, therapists neglect their own needs and find themselves implicitly promising to meet needs they cannot fulfill. In the long run, limits are as important as flexibility to establish a safe therapeutic environment, and to make clear what is necessary to live in the real world.

Case illustration

An experienced therapist, who prided himself on being able to meet even the extreme needs of his patients, became involved in the treatment of several patients with a history of sexual abuse. As a successful product of medical education and training, the therapist had taken on the belief that he should be able to respond at any hour, day or night, even at the cost of his sleep, health, mental stability, and family. He soon began to find himself awakened regularly at night, often being asked to engage in long discussions around the issue of suicide. He learned to dread the ring of the telephone and slept poorly, expecting to be awakened. The introduction of a new puppy into his household, and the responsibility of getting up at dawn's first light to walk the puppy, brought him to the brink of exhaustion. Violating his teachings not to talk to his patients about his own needs, the therapist told each of his patients that he retired early and that he expected each of them to respect his needs. Although he made it clear that he was available for serious emergencies, he also emphasized that he did not enjoy late night calls and would be much more capable of helping patients during office hours. After a stormy period of protest and rage on the part of his patients, evening and night calls decreased dramatically to only one or two calls every month. One of his patients later explored how she was acting out her anger by sadistically calling him repeatedly at home.

Trap #5: responsibility

The initial contract for psychotherapy (either explicit or implied) between patient and therapist involves a mutual agreement to pursue treatment which might eventually result in a positive benefit to the patient. As the therapy proceeds, however, this situation often becomes less clear. The therapy itself is arduous for the patient, involving extending trust which appears to be an invitation to be hurt. It also involves the uncovering and reliving of traumatic experiences which at times is overwhelming and intolerable. As a result, patients may wish to flee, either through leaving therapy completely or even through suicide. At such times the locus of the responsibility for the treatment seems to shift from a mutually held responsibility to being the therapist's responsibility. Therapists often find themselves in the position of urging patients to stay in treatment, or trying to convince patients not kill themselves. To these kinds of interventions patients frequently respond with logical sounding and compelling reasons as to why they should leave treatment or suicide. These situations leave therapists in untenable therapeutic positions where they seem to have the full responsibility of the patient's life and continued treatment. Moreover, in these kind of situations, the patient does not have to deal with her own ambivalence about the treatment. Since the therapist maintains the positive stance, the patient is actually more freed up to be more negative. Langs (1973) argues that even slight changes in the therapeutic contract are harmful to the therapy; in actual clinical practice, the therapeutic contract evolves along with the therapy, but certain basic tenets must remain. While therapists must empathize with the patient's experience of the difficulty of the therapy, they must also frequently clarify the nature of the therapy and the sharing of the responsibility for the work. Although it is sometimes the therapist's position of needing to be the one who maintains hope and to preserve the patients safety, therapists must also understand the need to step back and allow their patients to assume their share of the responsibility for their treatment and well-being.

Case illustration

About six months into the therapy of a young woman who had been brutally sexually abused as a child, the patient became very angry with her therapist at what she saw as an intrusive and unempathic remark. She fired her therapist who (probably correctly) insisted that she continue her therapy with him. She refused to come to appointments, at which point the therapist began calling her repeatedly at home and sometimes prior to her appointment times reminding her that she was to see him. The patient began angrily telling her therapist that she wanted to kill herself and that he could not prevent her. She convincingly argued that every day of her life involved great emotional pain, and if he really wanted to help that he would help her die. The therapist, who was feeling frustrated and confused, secretly wondered whether the patient was correct. He could easily see that the patient was leading a tortured existence, and wondered whether he should hospitalize her. Following consultation with a colleague, the therapist finally had a session with the patient in which he explored her choices about treatment. He explained that if necessary that he would take measures to keep her safe, but ultimately it was her choice whether or not to be in treatment with him, or even to be alive. He pointed out that it seemed that he was in the position of trying to persuade her to live, whereas the original agreement was to work on ways she could improve her life and not to kill herself. Following this discussion the patient appeared to be slightly calmer, and was able to talk about how trapped she felt in the relationship, which mirrored previous abusive relationships. The therapy continued on from that point.

Trap #6: control

Patients with a traumatic past, including those with histories of severe childhood abuse, exhibit the biphasic response described by investigators of post-traumatic stress disorder (Horowitz, 1976). Van der Kolk (1987, p.3) describes this biphasic response as "intrusive responses [consisting of] hyperactivity, explosive aggressive outbursts, startle responses, intrusive recollections in the form of nightmares and flashbacks, and reenactment of situations reminiscent of the trauma," alternating with the "numbing response [consisting] of emotional constriction, social isolation, retreat from family obligations, anhedonia, and a sense of estrangement." In other words, many patients seem to alternatively exist in either states of overwhelming loss of control or of attempting to maintain rigid control of themselves and their feelings, much like a light switch being turned on or off. It seems that having been in the position of being powerless in the face of abuse, and having been controlled by abusive figures, that these patients often attempt to take rigid control of their own lives and attempt to control events around them. However, given these patients' internal instability and their maladaptive self-reliance, this control is tenuous and frequently breaks down, resulting in periods of loss of control and inability to regain control, much to the frustration of their therapists. The knowledgeable therapist insists that some measure of control be let go in ways that can be productive, and does not accept long periods of the patient being sealed over as being inevitable. Similarly, therapists should not be in the position of tolerating endless flashbacks, and should make realistic demands for the patient to control these episodes. Often it later appears that the patient consciously or unconsciously arranges the circumstances to allow the flashbacks to continue, which relieves internal pressures for a time, but does not result in true abreaction or integration of the experiences. Although overcontrol and loss of control are inherent in the experience of traumatized patients, therapists need to push for increased ability to both let down control and to be in control, as a major goal of the treatment.

Case illustration

Even following many months of treatment, a patient continued to have long periods during which she distanced herself from her therapist, punctuated by episodes where she was out of control for long periods, having flashbacks of past traumatic experiences and becoming extremely regressed. These episodes resulted in long sessions often lasting two hours or more in the therapist's office, or the therapist being called to the patient's home for episodes which often extended into the early hours of the morning. Often the episodes were without clear therapeutic value, as the flashbacks were far too much for the patient to integrate, and thus were merely re-repressed. It also appeared that the patient was extending the episodes, insisting on poor lighting, avoiding eye contact, and refusing to focus on the real and present environment. After discussing the situation with the patient, the therapist began insisting that the flashback experiences be stopped after a short period of time, and that the patient use techniques that would achieve some sense of control. The patient readily admitted that she avoided having abreactive experiences in general, but when flashbacks finally occurred, she prolonged them, feeling that this would enable her to go for another long period of time without such experiences.

Trap #7: denial

Denial is a core defense for patients with a history of trauma. The need to believe that certain experiences did not occur, or that certain affects are not present, leads to the use of repression and dissociation. Collusion with patients' denial is a dangerous trap in treating traumatized patients. A long tradition of professional and social denial of the existence of child abuse and its long term sequelae (Goodwin, 1985; Masson, 1984) has encouraged such collusion, to the detriment of patients. Goodwin (1985), in discussing professional incredulity about multiple personality patients and child abuse, writes:

> When professionals join the family in insisting that nothing happened...dissociative defenses are strengthened... We observe, in interactions with patients with multiple personality disorder and abused children and their families, a shared negative hallucination... The multiple personality patient and the physician cling to the series of false symptoms and false diagnoses in proportion to their mutual need to blot out the reality of the multiplicity, and to blot out the unbearable experiences of real pain that triggered it (p.13–14).

Collusion in denying the often horrifying abusive backgrounds of traumatized patients makes it impossible to begin to address these experiences and eventually to neutralize them. Patients often convincingly argue that they have imagined stories about their pasts. Although this does occur (rarely), such statements must be reviewed skeptically since it is a good deal more common for patients to fabricate stories about good upbringings and uneventful childhoods, rather than to admit that their parents abused them (Goodwin *et al.*, 1979). Similarly, patients may acknowledge the history of trauma or abuse, but deny its significance (Chu, 1987). They may convincingly argue that they are aware of what happened to them and that they have worked such experiences through. However, the therapist must clearly examine whether the patient has affective understanding of the traumatic experiences and has thus worked them through, or whether the patient has only cognitive memories of the traumas and continues to be vulnerable to the re-emergence of the old affect. In any instance where the therapist colludes with denial on the part of the patient, there is likely to be a non-therapeutic, and perhaps dangerous, outcome.

Case illustration

Early in the therapy of a patient with suspected multiple personality disorder, a therapist began hearing about vague memories of physical and sexual abuse in childhood. Angry and tearful personalities appeared and began relating details of the abuse which was reported to have been sadistic and persisted over years. The therapist listened sympathetically to the story, but retained a healthy degree of skepticism. He interviewed the patient's father, the alleged abuser and a respected minister in his town church, who emphatically denied any abuse, and informed the therapist that the patient was a liar even as a child. In a subsequent discussion with the patient, the patient stated that she had lied about the abuse to get attention from the therapist and had faked multiple personalities. She proceeded to talk about her father's good qualities as a minister and parent, and was remorseful about maligning such an innocent person. The therapist, feeling vastly relieved of the burden of pursuing the issue of abuse any further, talked with the patient about the necessity of getting attention for positive actions rather than through false accusations. The patient was subsequently not prepared for a visit home to her father where she was attacked and raped, which was confirmed by medical examination.

Trap #8: projection

The traumatized patient defends against intolerable experiences, conflicts, and affects by disavowing them. Through dissociation and personality fragmentation, these phenomena can be owned by different parts of the self, or can be projected onto the external environment. Although most extreme in the case of multiple personality disorder, the internal world of many traumatized patients is conflicted and fragmented. The resolution of internal conflicts involves the exploration of their genesis in childhood trauma and abuse, and it is far easier for the patient to see the external world as a projection of the internal fragmentation. Thus, the therapist becomes the object of many confusing transferences (Wilbur, 1984, 1986). He or she is alternately seen as nurturing, abusive, friendly, hostile, empathic, cold, etc. The patient's inability to confront what is seen as intolerable and unbearable frequently results in an inability to make progress in treatment, but it is the therapist who is blamed for not being enough, not knowing enough, or not doing enough. The experience of being regarded in so many different ways (sometimes even in the course of a single hour), and the patient's tendency to blame the therapist provokes a wide variety of feelings and responses in therapists. Therapists must avoid acting out their own feelings such as anger or sadism, and must understand and interpret the transference. Therapists must also avoid colluding with the resistance, since this will lead to both patient and therapist becoming immobilized and blaming the therapist. Hospitalization of these patients usually raises even more confusion, as various staff members may become the object of projections, with some staff being regarded as nurturing, good, and helpful, and other staff being seen as insensitive, rigid, and incompetent. Combined with the inevitable struggles over control, the tendency of these patients to project can make inpatient hospitalizations major battles rather than helpful experiences.

Case illustration

During a period of patient's panic, her therapist made a comment which reflected some of the therapist's own experience, and which she felt the patient would see as comforting and empathic. To her surprise, the patient became furious and subsequently escalated to the point of requiring hospitalization. In the hospital, the patient began complaining that the staff were "on power trips" and attempting to control her. She claimed that certain staff members were inconsistent with one another, and that some staff members were hostile and abusive with her. The therapist met with the staff, who, in reality, were frustrated and angry at the patient and each other. She helped the staff understand that they were reacting to the patient's view of them as projections of her own internal chaos and ambivalence, and suggested a structure of non-punitive symptom control and work around aftercare issues. She then met with the patient, urging her to explore reasons for hospitalization rather than becoming side-tracked in battles with the staff. After a number of supportive interpretations about the patient's need to see the external world in conflict rather than to deal with her own internal conflicts, the patient was able to talk about how much the therapist became too close with her empathic comments, and how such intimacy became enormously threatening and intrusive in view of past abusive experiences. She spoke of how it was easier to distance through anger, seeing the therapist as violating her privacy, rather than to deal with past experiences, which led her to remain isolated.

Trap #9: idealization

There are few therapists who are not gratified by their patients regarding them as sensitive, clever, knowledgeable, and superior in their abilities. The trap is to believe that this represents the sum total of the patient's view of the therapist. As discussed in the trap of projection, the idealized transference is only one of the fragmented ways that the patient sees the therapist (Wilbur, 1984). The naive therapist can easily ignore the negative transferences, and can find himself or herself angry and confused when treated as a hostile abuser. An even

more unfortunate scenario occurs when both patient and therapist unconsciously collude to avoid the negative transference, often leading to
self-destructive activity, and not allowing for the resolution of the inevitable
hostility and rage which result from abuse. Ambivalence about others,
including the therapist, is a hallmark of traumatized patients; after all, such
patients lack an integrated sense of themselves, and hence see others in a variety
of fragmented and divergent ways. Therapists need to have a healthy sense of
self-awareness as to who and what they are, in order to keep their heads in the
shifting of transferences as presented by their patients. One particular form of
idealized transference, the eroticized transference, is particularly difficult. The
intense dependency of the patient is often reflected in the intensity of the
eroticized feelings, and therapists must be aware of the underlying ambivalence
in the relationship, as well as any resistances which are hidden behind
sexualized or romantic feelings (Wilbur, 1984).

Case illustration

A bright and articulate patient began in therapy by discussing the ignorance
and rigidity of her previous therapist. To the therapist it did seem as though the
previous therapist was not sensitive to the patient's needs, and he felt flattered
by the comparison. As the therapy progressed, the patient complimented the
therapist on his expert handling of various situations, leaving him enormously
gratified. After several months of more or less harmonious work, the patient
finally revealed that she was in love with her therapist, and felt that he was the
only one who would ever be able to understand her and her needs. The
therapist, who was unaware of concurrent negative transferences, felt quite
uncomfortable with this situation, viewing it as an unfortunate result of the
patient's responding to his warm and appealing personality. He responded that
he did not feel the same way about the patient, which resulted in the patient's
becoming enraged and reorganizing the office furniture. She later called the
therapist letting him know that she intended to kill herself since there was no
hope of ever having the therapist the way she wanted. After consultation, the
therapist began to explain transference to the patient, and to explore the full
range of her feelings towards him. The angry and self-destructive behavior
subsided somewhat, although the patient continued to feel "stupid" for having
revealed her feelings to her therapist. On the other hand, the patient began to
understand how her insecurities focused her needs and affections on her
therapist.

Trap #10: motivation

Given the extreme emotional pain that is often a part of the therapy of patients with abusive pasts, it often seems quite remarkable that patients can tolerate their own treatment. Certainly, the nature and amount of past abuse (and the corresponding level of disturbance) influence the eventual therapeutic outcome; in some instances, the psychological damage done by repeated and pervasive trauma is simply too much to repair. However, such factors as ego strength, ability to maintain even a conflicted relationship, and motivation play major roles in determining the outcome of treatment. The presence of ingrained severe character pathology, marked rigidity in coping mechanisms, or insufficient motivation suggests a poorer prognosis. Motivation is a complex phenomenon, and is certainly influenced by both the patient's internal characteristics and the external environment. For example, a history of personal failures leading to a strong belief of one's inability to change, the necessity for maintaining functional ability, or the need to maintain crucial relationships may all impact on the amount of motivation that the patient brings to the therapy. For most patients, motivation is assessed by actions and behaviors over time. Although it is usually difficult to assess progress over a few weeks or months, it is realistic to expect overall forward motion over several months. Verbalization is much less reliable than behavior. All patients verbalize ambivalence about the therapy. Some move on while others seem to have the conscious or unconscious goal of maintaining the status quo. Such "stuck" patients may verbalize a wish for progress but may actually only use the therapist as an ego resource for coping with reality. Therapists need to be aware that patients vary widely in their motivation and ability to improve, and it is prudent to set realistic goals. Not all patients are interested in resolving past events or in personality change and integration, and it is certainly acceptable to help a patient achieve some level of stability and more harmonious functioning and relationships.

Case illustration

Following three years of individual psychotherapy with a competent and experienced therapist, a young woman seemed to be more stable. The therapy had consisted of individual psychotherapy up to three times a week, and intermittent hospitalizations for suicidality, including one admission of over a year. Although the patient continued to verbalize that she wished to understand past traumatic events, she continued to resist dealing with her past in many different ways. Following confrontation about her resistance, the patient reluctantly admitted that she felt she couldn't tolerate the feelings which accompanied the discussion of old traumas. She felt that her ultimate goal was simply to find people to be sensitive to her needs and to take care of her. She expressed little or no interest in independent functioning. She was fearful of exploratory psycho-therapy but felt compelled to say that she wanted to pursue it in order to please her therapist. She also feared that any progress she made would result in aban-donment by the therapist. The therapist and patient agreed that they would limit the goals of treatment, and would have an on-going relationship based on supportive interventions to help the patient function better in her life. The therapist also felt that therapy with him, a man, might have been making the therapy more difficult and suggested that the patient add a women's support group. With these changes, the treatment appeared to proceed with fewer self-sabotaging activities and more obvious signs of progress.

CONCLUSION

Traps, binds, dilemmas, and conflicts in treatment are common in the psychotherapies of many conditions, but seem to have an added drama in the intense relationship between therapist and trauma survivor. Patients who are trauma survivors present with a variety of resistances including reluctance to wrestle with the abusive experiences, the inability to adequately trust the therapist, and the inability to draw on memories. Therapists respond in a variety of ways based on their level of skill and experience, and on their countertransference and counterresistance. Experience and understanding do tend to reduce the anxiety inherent in these situations, but even experienced therapists find themselves in treatment traps, as they are an intrinsic part of the therapy of traumatized patients.

The case illustrations and discussions of treatment traps are self-explana-tory. This paper is not intended to cover all treatment traps or to establish rules for what to do, or not to do, in any particular situation. Rather, the paper is designed to encourage therapists to be thoughtful in making decisions through understanding the dynamics of the treatment arena. Finding a balance in such issues as flexibility versus limits, acceptance versus confrontation, or even the patient's versus the therapist's needs, are all part of the skill, judgement, and art of psychotherapy. Finally, it is important to realize that the issues raised in this paper are core issues in the treatment itself, and how they are managed is a crucial part of the therapeutic process. Knowledge, understanding, patience and compassion on the part of the therapist will enhance the therapeutic process, and may make it more productive for the patient and therapist.

REFERENCES

Braun, E.G. (1986) 'Issues in the psychotherapy of multiple personality disorder.' In B.C. Braun, (ed.) *Treatment of multiple personality disorder.* Washington, DC: American Psychiatric Press.

Bryer, J.B., Nelson, B.A., Miller, J.B. and Krol, P.A. (1987) Childhood sexual and physical abuse as factors in adult psychiatric illness. *American Journal of Psychiatry,* 144(11), 1426–1430.

Chessick, R.D. (1982) Current issues in intensive psychotherapy. *American Journal of Psychotherapy,* 36, 438–449.

Chu, J.A. (1987) The repetition compulsion revisited: Reliving dissociated trauma. Paper presented at the Fourth International Conference on Multiple Personality/Dissociative States, Chicago.

Chu, J.A. (1988) Some aspects of resistance in the treatment of multiple personality disorder. *Dissociation,* 1(2), 34–38.

Finkelhor, D. (1984) *Child sexual abuse: New theory and research.* New York: Free Press.

Glover, E. (1955) *The technique of psychoanalysis.* New York: International Universities Press.

Goodwin, J. (1985) 'Credibility problems in multiple personality disorder and abused children.' In P.P. Kluft, (ed.) *Childhood antecedents of multiple personality disorder.* Washington, DC: American Psychiatric Press.

Goodwin, J., Sahd, D. and Rada, R. (1979) Incest hoax: False accusations, false denials. *Bulletin of the American Academy of Psychiatry and the Law,* 6, 269–276.

Greenson, R. (1967) *The technique and practice of psychoanalysis.* New York: International Universities Press.

Herman, J. (1981) *Father-daughter incest.* Cambridge: Harvard University Press.

Horowitz, M.J. (1976) *Stress response syndromes.* New York: Jason Aronson.

Kluft, R.P. (1984) Aspects of the treatment of multiple personality disorder. *Psychiatric Annals,* 14(1), 51–55.

Langs, R. (1973) *The techniques of psychoanalytic psychotherapy (Vol. 1).* New York: Jason Aronson.

Langs, R. (1981) *Resistance and interventions.* New York: Jason Aronson.

Masson, J.M. (1984) *The assault on the truth: Freud's suppression of the seduction theory.* New York: Farrar, Straus and Giroux.

Mays, D.T. and Franks, C.M. (1985) *Negative outcome in psychotherapy and what to do about it.* New York: Springer Publishing Company.

Richert, A. (1983) Differential prescription for psychotherapy on the basis of client role preferences. *Psychotherapy: Theory, research and practice,* 20, 321–329.

Russell, D.E.H. (1986) *The secret trauma: Incest in the lives of girls and women.* New York: Basic Books.

Spiegel, D. (1986) 'Dissociation, double binds, and the posttraumatic stress in multiple personality disorder.' In B.G. Braun, (ed.) *Treatment of multiple personality disorder.* Washington DC: American Psychiatric Press.

Strean, H.S. (1985) *Resolving resistances in psychotherapy.* New York: Joseph Wiley and Sons.

Van der Kolk, B.A. (1987) 'The psychological consequences of overwhelming life experiences.' In B.A. van der Kolk, (ed.) *Psychological Trauma.* Washington, DC: American Psychiatric Press.

Wilbur, C.B. (1984) Treatment of multiple personality. *Psychiatric Annals,* 14(1), 27–31.

Wilbur, C.B. (1986) 'Psychoanalysis and multiple personality disorder.' In B.G. Braun, (ed.) *Treatment of multiple personality disorder.* Washington, DC: American Psychiatric Press.

Winnicott, D. (1965) *The maturational process and the facilitating environment.* New York: International Universities Press.

15

Severe Personality Disorder Patients: Treatment Issues and Selection for In-patient Psychotherapy*

Kingsley Norton and R.D. Hinshelwood
1996

. . . .

Editors' reflections

The following paper highlights the challenges which many services face when offering treatment for personality disorder. The diagnosis and/or severity of a personality disorder invariably does not assist us in establishing treatment plans or prognosis. The authors promote services adopting a stance of 'enquiry and understanding' rather than becoming caught in dominance and control dynamics. They also highlight the importance of setting achievable treatment goals which have a 'here and now' quality rather than focusing upon future goals which, for the service user, feel beyond their current capabilities. The authors make an argument for specialist services but also for greater sharing of skills, knowledge and communication between different services.

. . . .

*   Originally published in *British Journal of Psychiatry*, *168*, 723–731. Reprinted here by permission of The Royal College of Psychiatrists.

Abstract

Background. *Severe personality disorder (SPD) is an imprecise but useful term refer-ring to some notoriously difficult to treat psychiatric patients. Their long-term psychi-atric treatment is often unsuccessful, in spite of hospitalisation. The specialist expertise of in-patient psychotherapy units (IPUs) can successfully meet some of SPD patients' needs.*

Method. *Relevant literature on the subject is summarised and integrated with the authors' specialist clinical experience.*

Results. *Many clinical problems with SPD patients are interpersonal and prevent any effective therapeutic alliance, which is necessary for successful treatment. With in-patients, inconsistencies in treatment delivery and issues surrounding compulsory treatment reinforce patients' mistrust of professionals, compromising accurate diagnosis and an assessment of the need for specialist IPU referral.*

Conclusions. *General psychiatric teams are well-placed to plan long-term treatment for SPD patients which may include IPU treatment. Timely referral of selected SPD patients to an IPU maximises a successful outcome, especially if there is appropriate post-discharge collaboration with general psychiatric teams to consolidate gains made.*

Severe personality disorder (SPD) occurs in approximately 4% of the adult pop-ulation (Casey, 1988). It is an imprecise but useful clinical term (Kernberg, 1984). Patients in this category make extensive use of the health services, social services and other agencies, often with little lasting benefit. A diagnosis of SPD tends to worsen the prognosis of a co-existing symptom disorder, whether psychotic or non-psychotic (Tyrer, 1988). A worse prognosis may apply to a co-existing physical disorder, because of the difficulty many personality disor-dered patients have in generally playing their role as patient and complying with treatment requirements (Norton and Smith, 1994). SPD is also associated with many of the target areas in the *Health of the Nation* document (DoH, 1992): unhealthy eating and drinking habits; smoking; increased 'accidents'; Human immunodeficiency virus (HIV)/Acquired immunodeficiency syndrome (AIDS); other mental illness and suicide (Norton, 1992*a*).

INTERPERSONAL PROBLEMS

The trademark of SPD patients is an impairment of their interpersonal and social functioning. This makes it difficult to engage many of them in treatment since the clinical encounter with them is frequently marked by negative feelings, both in them but also in the staff involved in treatment. Intense hostile or controlling reactions in the latter serve to perpetuate or aggravate an aggressive, or passive-aggressive, response from patients. In this way, unhelpful cycles of maladaptive interpersonal functioning are set up which undermine any collaborative approach to treatment or even entering into a therapeutic alliance, which could support the achievement of mutually agreed and relevant clinical goals.

Pines (1978) makes the point in the context of out-patient group psychotherapy:

> Those attending personality disorder patients, feel impelled to conform to a pattern imposed by the patient, so that we begin to feel provoked, hostile, persecuted and (have) to behave exactly as the patients need us to, becoming rejecting and hostile!.

This phenomenon applies equally to staff working in in-patient settings where they are in enduring contact throughout the day and night with such patients and are propelled with even more force, than in out-patient therapy, into these mutually hostile and rejecting interactive patterns.

The implicit demands (for example, to follow medical advice involving lifestyle changes as in relinquishing 'action' solutions to emotional distress or conflict) made on SPD patients by conventional medical and psychiatric treatment can render them unhelpable by expecting more from them than they can deliver. This can then rebound negatively on medical and other staff who become embattled and disillusioned. Well-intentioned helpers become frustrated and then sometimes unhelpful and negative. As a result, many SPD patients do not receive planned or coordinated treatment. Hospitalisation, to a general psychiatric unit, is often considered only in the midst of a crisis or some medical or psychiatric emergency and seldom as a planned measure and as part of an overall treatment strategy. Whatever treatment is planned it is important for staff to be aware that the setting of realistic and achievable goals is crucially important, since with many SPD patients even apparently trivial treatment 'failures' may bring about a complete breakdown in the therapeutic alliance.

VICTIM AND PERPETRATOR

In traditional psychiatric in-patient settings, SPD patients may find interpersonal reward for their maladaptive behaviour or 'action' solutions, such as overdosing or self-mutilation. Damage to self, others or property often results in more intensive interpersonal attention or contact in the form of additional nursing supervision, so-called 'specialling'. In such a circumstance the patient is implicitly viewed as incapable of accepting responsibility for his or her actions, and as a victim of his or her condition. Such endorsement of maladaptive behaviour maintains the status quo of the patient, in relation to the setting, by precluding any relevant questioning which might lead to an alteration of their ingrained maladaptive attitudes and thereby permit personality maturation. In other instances, equally untherapeutic, the patient may be held as if totally responsible, as the perpetrator of any damage, and then reprimanded and/or discharged from the hospital. Staff may alternately strive to persuade the same patient to stay in hospital for treatment – as victim – or else to exhort them to leave – as perpetrator.

A partial view of the SPD patient, as either a victim or a perpetrator, is inevitably a distorted and one-sided perspective. If staff reflect only this back, the patient does not have to consider being both victim *and* perpetrator and therefore no novel questions about the self (or, implicitly, about others) are raised. Narrow or extreme institutional responses, which reinforce 'either/or' thinking, remove any opportunity for the patient to learn from experience (Norton and Dolan, 1995a).

SPD patients create mutual hostility between themselves and their carers, but also hostile divisions among the staff involved with their treatment. In a classic paper, Main (1957) describes the way some patients cling to and use their 'ailment', as an instrument for managing good and bad relationships alternately with different members of staff. The 'good' relationship often incorporates the patient as victim, and the 'bad', as perpetrator. The different staff involved tend to occupy the complementary roles of kind defender and of cruel attacker. Kind defenders and cruel attackers do not see eye to eye, hence the formation of a pattern of patient-generated 'splitting' in staff teams, albeit usually along pre-existing 'fault lines' in the staff team. The phenomenon has been noted by others (Stanton and Schwartz, 1954) and its effect is to impair the quality of treatment provided by staff, through the destructive effect of their own disagreements. Sometimes the latter are covert or otherwise ignored but this only leads to more difficulties with providing consistent and coordinated treatment.

To change this state of affairs, in-patient staff need to achieve and communicate a more complex and impartial view of their patients. Patients are neither simply victims nor simply perpetrators and, through therapy, they need to develop capacities to identify accurately both aggressive and vulnerable aspects of their personalities. This is an arduous process, both for the individual patient (since, at least temporarily, the patient feels more conflicted) and for the institution and its staff. Thus, staff bear the brunt of the patient's familiar maladaptive ways of dealing with unbearable conflict, (often via aggressive 'acting-out'), and also their high levels of distress once the conflict is owned and located intrapersonally (revealed by the dismantling of ingrained defensive strategies). Both sorts of behaviour and expressions of conflict can be difficult to cope with, especially where there is oscillation (sometimes rapid) between the two.

IN-PATIENT PSYCHOTHERAPY UNITS

IPUs have been classified in a number of ways. Hinshelwood (1988) describes three main types: (1) psychotherapy is only part of the therapeutic armoury of the psychiatric unit run on conventional hospital lines; (2) formal psychotherapy takes place within a special milieu which is designed to support and complement it; and (3) psychotherapy and sociotherapy are integrated with the primary focus being on the unit as a whole. For the purpose of this paper, the focus is on types (2) and (3); in the absence of firm or definite criteria to distinguish them, they will be considered as a single category called IPU.

Over the last 50 years, IPUs have developed treatment methods which rely on the creation of a culture of enquiry, or reflective practice, for their therapeutic efficacy. All aspects and assumptions of the culture and activity of the Unit are open to question, while the structure and boundaries are maintained as strictly invariant. This shift in the total orientation of the Unit is required to avoid extreme and polarised views about their patients' maladaptive behaviour or other expressions of conflict and to minimise the impact of SPD patient-generated 'splits' in the IPU's staff team. This is needed to support and foster the patients' adaptive behaviour (especially their capacity to experience and show vulnerability) and concomitantly to challenge and question their maladaptive attitudes and behaviour (Jones, 1952; Main, 1983). The aim of specialist in-patient psychotherapy, as in the therapeutic community, is to establish an environment and atmosphere that embodies a 'culture of enquiry' (Main, 1983; Norton, 1992b) within a predictably structured environment, since this can enable some SPD patients to feel safe and secure, i.e. emotionally contained.

The IPU emphasis is on questioning and understanding rather than blaming and punishing. Its goal is to avoid the extreme positions of responding to the patient in an 'either/or' fashion – either as victim or as perpetrator. However, this is difficult to achieve since treatment needs to be built on a foundation of accurate empathic connection with the patient. (In many IPUs the patient's peer group contributes actively to make an empathic contact and to engage the patient in a therapeutic alliance.) The above combined approach can facilitate some SPD patients to move from being 'actors' to becoming 'thinkers and feelers' (Masterson, 1972). The latter achievement can be seen to represent the internalisation by the patient of important aspects of the structure and pervading culture of the hospital. In avoiding a blaming, punishing and shaming response, the Unit presents SPD patients with an unfamiliar situation which calls from them a new and more thoughtful posture, if they are to flourish in this environment. They learn, as a direct consequence, to start to question and understand themselves rather than to perpetuate an internal self-punitive relationship with themselves.

IPUs must ensure a well-serviced and coherent (external) organisational structure, since SPD patients do not have an adequate (internal) mental structure (Greene and Johnson, 1987). Crucial to this work is effective communication between staff throughout the 24 hours (from day to night to day). Meticulous attention is paid to staff's mutual support and self-examination in order to confront and 'metabolise' the problematic emotional responses engendered by SPD patients. Otherwise, unhelpfully prolonged polarisation and splitting of staff attitudes and beliefs (both in respect of their patients and one another) arise. Entrenched contradictory views of the patient, for example victim or perpetrator, remain unspoken and unresolved with eventual demoralisation and possibly hostile acting-out by the staff against each other or the Unit. Each IPU has its own organisational solution to this central problem of how to optimise communication and maintain a therapeutic culture which affords emotional as well as physical containment.

At the Cassel Hospital continual enquiry informs a detailed scrutiny of the relationship between the key nurse and the individual psychotherapist (James, 1986). Supervision of this dyad teases out the subtle tensions between these two important staff (Tischler, 1986). Incompatibilities or irregularities can be important representations of the patient's inner world. At the same time such examination starts an exploration of the higher order system of the whole therapeutic community; as well as the possibility of the patient's internalisation of the world outside him or her in a creative integration of it with his or her own psychic world. At the Henderson Hospital, regular and frequent meetings of the whole staff team throughout the day maximise effective communication, especially between staff during 'after-groups'. Therein, immediately, any differences of perspective on the group are exposed and staff challenge one another's perceptions, technique and formulations; as well as providing each other with mutual support. The aim is to integrate or resolve contradictory views of patients as individuals and as a group. There is formal supervision of the staff group itself and a sensitivity group which is facilitated by an outside therapist, to further examine the ramifications of such aspects.

INDICATIONS FOR IPU REFERRAL

The question of which patients, and when, to admit to an IPU faces many professionals working in psychiatry and in other disciplines. Assessing suitability requires knowledge of both the patient and the particular IPU. Obtaining information about the latter should be straightforward; it is the patient who is difficult to know. Because of the inherent difficulties of forging a treatment alliance with SPD patients, however, the validity of the diagnostic assessment may be low because of limited compliance or cooperation. Even so, patients admitted to IPUs tend to have many features of history, mental state and level of current psychosocial functioning in common. As such, the latter may be relevant indications for considering IPU referral, even if the precise PD or SPD diagnostic label is difficult to apply with confidence.

History

Most SPD patients have histories of serious physical and/or sexual abuse or neglect in their formative years and in relation to their parents or substitute carers. The disorganised and insecure attachment patterns which are established yield concomitant internal working models which are reflected in, and perpetuated by, impaired attachment patterns to others later on, in adolescence and adulthood.

Many SPD patients come into contact with social, penal and probation services. Even those with no formal forensic history often provide a history of serious anti-social behaviour or of committing a crime which has gone undetected. Sometimes the lack of detection is because such behaviour comes under the heading of 'domestic violence'. Where such anti-social histories are present, evidence of a disordered personality or disordered earlier development is often traceable, more or less continuously, back into childhood. Such information is only elicited, however, if routine history-taking covers all relevant areas of enquiry.

Most SPD patients suitable for in-patient psychotherapy have not benefited from repeated short-term hospitalisations in general psychiatric wards or from a range of out-patient treatments. They show an accumulating number of failed relationships and poor occupational records and evidence that hopelessness and destructive living styles have become incorporated into the personality (Greben, 1983). Many such patients are referred as a 'last resort' testifying to the failure of other treatment approaches and to the entrenched and serious nature of the psychopathology and interpersonal difficulties.

Some characteristics of SPD patients at presentation to in-patient psychotherapy have prognostic value and can serve as clinical indicators for admission.

Basic educational achievement, perhaps only a solitary examination pass, may represent a sign of a capacity to commit to a period of study – it is the capacity for commitment which may augur well for treatment. (Obviously innate talent and high intelligence can confound this conclusion.) A period of stable work can likewise represent a personality strength as can the maintenance of some interpersonal stability, for example maintaining a close intimate relationship for more than six months (Whiteley, 1970). SPD patients' recall of a positive relationship in childhood may also be prognostically important (Healey and Kennedy, 1993).

Mental state examination

Positive psychotic symptoms or prominent negative symptomatology, associated with psychosis, are usually contraindications to intensive in-patient psychotherapy. Likewise a significant learning disability will usually mean that the patient will not be accepted, principally because they are not able to function psychosocially at a level equal to that of other patients. They consequently risk becoming scapegoated and thereby unable to benefit from the positive aspects of membership of a cohesive patient peer group. Motivation for change must be present. This usually requires informal patient status. Assessing motivation may be difficult when there are outstanding court cases or formal patient status prevails, since acceptance for treatment may have implications for the courts, as an alternative disposal to imprisonment, or for the relaxation of formal treatment conditions. Patients' acknowledgement of some responsibility for their problems, especially where there is a history of violence, rather than a tendency to blame others is usually a positive indicator. Being able to identify emotional responses in themselves and to provide a 'cause-effect' account of themselves, whereby psychological consequences of their actions can be established, are good indicators for psychotherapy.

Diagnosis

There is no simple relationship between personality disorder diagnosis and in-patient psychotherapy even though there is evidence of a differential beneficial effect of dynamic psychotherapy according to PD diagnosis (Stone, 1993). Using DSM-III/IV classification of PD, it appears that Cluster B diagnoses are most responsive to dynamic psychotherapeutic approaches, this being the most common approach utilised within IPUs. Most SPD patients, however, have more than one PD subtype diagnosis and a single patient may have PD subtypes from more than one cluster, making it difficult to translate findings from the research literature directly into clinical practice.

The assessment of the severity of personality disorder is complex and no satisfactory and agreed method exists (Norton and Dolan, 1995b). Some argue that the number of personality disorder subtype diagnoses per patient is a marker of severity. The presence of more than one personality disorder diagnosis (Dolan *et al.*, 1995) therefore may indicate SPD and hence, on the grounds of severity, a patient who is appropriate for referral for in-patient psychotherapy. The relationship between severity of personality disorder and treatability, however, is not clear. Assessing the suitability of SPD patients for treatment in an IPU requires taking into account the factors already mentioned above.

The psychiatric literature is of little help in identifying precisely those who will benefit from in-patient psychotherapy. In practice, referrers often do not use ICD or DSM diagnostic PD categories but rather a variety of other 'labels': forensic cases; acting out patients; treatment-resistant cases; 'abusers' of various categories; those with serious eating disorders and service wasters. These descriptive categories obviously lack the precision and reliability of those from the standard classifications but they appear to have a currency and utility in everyday clinical practice. As such, the above may form useful guides to would-be referrers.

Dangerousness

Acute dangerousness has been suggested as a reason for considering in-patient psychotherapy for SPD patients (Knight, 1953). In this context, however, acute dangerousness has to be seen as existing alongside some positive indication for a psychological treatment intervention. This also has to be considered in the context of the particular IPU and the level of security which exists there. Dangerousness *per se* is no indication for treatment in an IPU (see above). However, dangerousness is not a fixed entity but reflects interactive aspects of the individual patient and the setting, importantly the patient's interpersonal environment. The degree of assessed dangerousness in some patients, therefore, can diminish with admission to an IPU because of the increased emotional containment available there. In such cases there is then less or no need for physical containment and for the use of tranquillising or sedative medication. In others, while the risk of dangerousness is diminished there is still a considerable risk of violence during treatment and medication is required in addition (see below). In some patients who are accepted for treatment, there is a need to negotiate an agreement with the referring psychiatric team, that they will accept back an SPD patient if tertiary in-patient therapy breaks down (see below).

Medication

Depending on the IPU, the continued need for psychotropic medication or the assessed high risks of discontinuing medication may represent contraindications for admission there. However, many SPD patients can only be managed with the use of psychotropic medication (Stein, 1992). IPUs differ in their policy, some allowing such prescriptions and others not. Overall, there tends to be an assumption that medication is reduced to a level at which patients can tolerate their symptoms while continuing therapy. As often as not the patient gains an enriched self-esteem if he or she is realistically able to forego, or lessen, dependence on medication. We need to recognise, too, that many who receive such medication, on conventional psychiatric units, would not need it (or not at such high levels) if the therapeutic environment contained them emotionally in a more effective way.

Staff in IPUs, as well as in other settings, need to be aware of the psychodynamic factors which influence prescribing practice, sometimes leading to over-medication or under-medicating. Thus: (1) Medication can represent a substitute gratification for unmet personal needs; (2) it can be used beneficially as a 'transitional object', even facilitating more mature relationships or substituting a form of dependence which is preferable to more destructive alternatives; (3) therapists and their SPD patients typically risk enacting 'master-slave' relationships, and using medication may increase the temptation for the therapist to act in an authoritarian way; (4) staff may 'resort' to medication when their own interpersonal resources are used up or to alleviate their own anxiety or indirectly express anger; (5) medication may become a non-verbal method of controlling feelings, contradicting for some the therapeutic goal of enabling patients to contain feelings in words (Miller, 1989). It is important that neither staff nor patients feel that the use of drugs is synonymous with the failure of psychological treatment approaches since there is evidence of a genuine synergistic effect which yields therapeutic results not available from either treatment ingredient alone.

IMPLICATIONS FOR GENERAL PSYCHIATRIC UNITS

The general acute psychiatric in-patient unit is not set up to deal with many of the specific treatment needs of SPD patients. Such units serve many purposes, and importantly a custodial and asylum function, for a comprehensive range of psychiatric diagnoses. The internal organisational structure and culture of the units reflects this. The style is characteristically authoritarian rather than democratic and the relationships which go on inside are often based rather more on dominance and control than on empathy and enquiry (see earlier). There is thus a tendency for ward staff to view patients in characteristically narrow ways, representing simple dichotomies. Patients are thus construed as sick (psychotic) or healthy (sane).

Many SPD patients are perceived as not sick and staff are then faced with a dilemma. If the patient is legitimately a patient but is not psychotic, hence not sick, yet is not healthy (otherwise they would not be in hospital) then what are they? If not healthy yet in hospital the other option tends to be to view the patient as 'bad'. Rationalisations for such perceived badness are not difficult to find since SPD patients are often willing partners and readily provide evidence of badness, whether in not playing the patient role appropriately (in being irresponsible and failing to take steps towards appropriate health care); in being self-destructive; or in being aggressive or violent to others or to property.

Very often SPD patients in such a setting are not willing participants in their treatment and the required therapeutic task, which would be to minimise the influence of the power dynamic and to engage the patients through facilitating an awareness of impediments to their forming a straightforward treatment alliance, is difficult to achieve. Staff need to be aware that active engagement in treatment cannot be taken for granted and they need to know what to do in order to foster this. In essence, they need to convey to the SPD patient: (1) An understanding of his or her difficulties in relating to others (especially those in social positions of power and authority); (2) that this difficulty is based upon low self-esteem, ambivalence, fear of intimacy and basic mistrust; (3) that these aspects may be understandable and of survival value to the patient given past experiences (although often at the cost of loneliness and a sense of profound alienation) but currently are largely maladaptive (Norton and Dolan, 1995a).

The SPD patient's successful engagement is a necessary prerequisite for successful treatment, whether psychiatric or psychotherapeutic. This necessary first stage, however, is often not achieved, especially in general psychiatric in-patient units. Hierarchical and authoritarian arrangements tend to serve to increase the likelihood of treatment difficulties, including violence (Powell et al., 1994). Victim-perpetrator dynamics are commonly observable and are based on a power differential between patients and their carers. The treatment situation serves to maintain a status quo since psychic tension is discharged more readily inter-personally between patient and staff (or staff and staff, as a result of 'splits') than it is contained intrapsychically by the patient and staff. For the patient, the potential for remembering rather than acting is lost and the experience is of custodial, rather than therapeutic, containment. Patients do not become thinkers and feelers (see above).

The difficulty facing many in-patient psychiatric units often becomes: (1) Effecting a swift response to patients' emotional needs which are expressed as 'actions' of one sort or another; (2) facilitating an environment which allows an examination of antecedents and consequences, close in time to the behaviour, thereby maximising new learning; (3) providing an emotional atmosphere which is empathic but which avoids simple condoning or condemning of maladaptive behaviour, which supports a victim-perpetrator dynamic; (4) providing human support systems as alternatives for discharging psychic tension and for dealing with more adaptively expressed distress; (5) formulating a treatment plan which incorporates the necessary range of therapeutic environments (including possible referral to an IPU) enabling movement from one to another consequent upon the patient progressing, for example from in-patient to day-patient status.

SPD patients are often chronically suicidal and, as such, they demand a particular, unrelenting vigilance from the staff. In-patient staff members can feel, and often are, loaded with the burden of predicting and averting the successful suicide. Repetitive threats of death with few actual occurrences produce, in staff, anxiety rather than a sense of mastery (Schwartz et al., 1974). Therefore, it is important for staff to have a realistic therapeutic contract and to feel they have a say in what is feasible. Patients still do commit suicide once hospitalised. Simple supervision without opportunities for confrontation and enquiry may only produce a therapeutic stalemate which, the longer it goes on, the more gloomy the prognosis becomes. Coming to terms with the realistic possibility of suicide, despite the staff's best efforts to prevent it, is one of the markers of a cohesive and mutually supportive staff team treating SPD patients. Strong suicidal ideation and suicidal activity are probably the commonest causes of severe disharmony in in-patient staff teams, save only for instances of successful suicide, serious physical injury or homicide.

CONCLUSIONS

Disadvantages of non-specialist in-patient units

Many SPD patients are admitted to acute psychiatric units even if this is not a planned measure but as a response to crisis. Often the occurrence is unwelcomed by both patient and in-patient staff, even though there may have been an initial experience of relief by the former. Sometimes the admission is part of a repeating pattern of admission and discharge, which is already associated with mutual frustration and pessimism.

In many instances the scene is set more as a battleground than as a fertile environment for treatment. Victim-perpetrator dynamics abound. Staff may see the same patient, at different times, as victim or perpetrator. The staff are often experienced by the SPD patient as being victimisers and indeed staff may feel this themselves, as when they are required to enforce treatment or prevent absconding. At other times, however, staff feel themselves the victims of both the patients and the psychiatric and legal system, in having to treat SPD patients at all. The victim-perpetrator split can also be played out entirely within the staff team, some staff feeling victimised by other staff, and even with each faction feeling victimised by the other.

In performing such complementary roles, in relation to their patients, some staff are more comfortable with one rather than the other pole. Oscillating between roles or occupying one or other polarities, as above, is draining of staff's personal resources and, ultimately, of morale. Individual staff members may be unable to divorce themselves from work issues, when not working, and have to rely on existing personal coping strategies and their own social networks for support. Both of these may be inadequate in relation to the large size of the task involved in looking after SPD patients on in-patient units.

Long-term treatment planning

In-patient admission of SPD patients, although often problematic, can be conceived as an opportunity. Admission offers the possibility of establishing a therapeutic alliance and, if appropriate, of forging a treatment contract with the patient which is sufficiently long-term and accurately tailored to the patients' particular needs. However, engagement in treatment is not once-and-for-all since it is readily undermined by both patient and staff factors. In the patient, it is basic mistrust in professionals, together with ambivalence about giving up familiar patterns of behaviour and accepting help, which dominate the clinical picture. On the side of the professionals, it is maintaining their integrity as a staff team (i.e. avoiding unduly prolonged or profound splits among themselves) and maintaining good communication in order to provide a consistent implementation of the treatment plan which is problematic. Special attention needs to be focused on these aspects surrounding admission, discharge or transfer to and from the in-patient unit. Ideally, such moves require joint planning with the relevant staff, including others from the previous or next treatment resource. Any move, ideally, should reflect a genuine change in a patient's clinical status and its timing discussed or negotiated with the patient, as far as this is appropriate. The general psychiatric team is often best placed to consider also the appropriateness of a referral to an IPU.

Advantages of the IPU

IPUs can select their SPD patients, aiming to admit only those who have a good prognosis. Patients form a more or less homogeneous diagnostic group, so a single model of treatment can suffice. The aims of treatment, for example to help patients to depend maturely on others rather than to resort to 'action' solutions of various kinds (including chemical dependence on drugs or alcohol) can be conveyed to all members of the staff team. Treatment strategies are established to ensure as consistent as possible a delivery of the treatment employed, through maximising good inter-staff communication and minimising the detrimental effects of the inevitable splitting processes. To support this, the usual staff–staff and staff–patient hierarchies are flattened.

IPU treatment, although complex, follows a protocol with which all staff can become readily familiar, there being no need to be acquainted with a vast range of treatments applicable to different diagnoses and clinical exigencies. Even so, the work is experienced as arduous since SPD patients, in striving to give up familiar, albeit maladaptive, patterns of dealing with internal conflict, experience and express more distress. The treatment therefore demands much of staff, especially since they are not protected by some of the usual staff–patient differences and usual degree of hierarchy in their relationships. There is thus a need for significant levels of staff support and supervision.

Collaboration between the IPU and the non-specialist in-patient unit

There are a number of points of collaboration between the IPU and other in-patient settings. The non-specialist unit can initiate contact by requesting an opinion on the current clinical management of an SPD patient *in situ* or by requesting an assessment for admission to the IPU. Meaningful engagement in treatment in the in-patient setting and/or the presence of a working therapeutic alliance may represent important indicators of suitability, other relevant criteria being present and there being no overriding contraindications.

The IPU staff may wish to involve the referring team in after-care, either handing it over completely or involving active collaboration. Alternatively, contact may be established simply to convey what the treatment plans post-discharge are. Ideally, IPUs are adequately resourced so that they can provide continuity of treatment post-discharge if this is clinically indicated. However, this is sometimes not the case or problematic for non-clinical reasons, for example, the long distance between a patient's usual residence and the location of the out-patient treatment. Peripatetic outreach teams can overcome this obstacle, but only to a limited extent. Since IPUs are rare, in the UK, geography is often a deciding factor in the provision and nature of the follow-up treatment.

IPU treatment is not always successful and failures may require emergency or planned transfer of an SPD patient from the IPU to another in-patient setting. Joint discussions can inform future management including an assessment of the need for compulsory treatment, higher levels of security, and/or the use of medication, as well as considering how any limited beneficial responses to the IPU can be translated into the non-specialist setting. It is also possible to discuss ways in which any previous adverse responses to the non-specialist in-patient setting can be minimised or avoided. Ideally, such dialogues take place outside of a 'crisis' situation since this maximises the chances of a successful exchange of views and minimises miscommunications or the development of unhealthy 'splits' between the specialist and general units.

ACKNOWLEDGEMENT

This paper is based on one presented by the authors at the Autumn 1994 Psychotherapy Section meeting of the Royal College of Psychiatrists.

REFERENCES

Casey, P. (1988) 'The epidemiology of personality disorder.' In P. Tyrer, ed. *Personality Disorder: Diagnosis, Management and Care.* London: Wright. p.74–81.

Department of Health (1992) *The Health of the Nation: A Strategy for Health in England.* London: HMSO (Cm 1985).

Dolan, B., Evans, C. and Norton, K.R.W. (1995) Multiple Axis-II diagnosis of personality disorder. *British Journal of Psychiatry,* 166, 107–112.

Greben, S. (1983) The multi-dimensional inpatient treatment of severe character disorders. *Canadian Journal of Psychiatry,* 28, 97–101.

Greene, L.R. and Johnson, D.R. (1987) Leadership and structuring of the large group. *International Journal of Therapeutic Communities,* 8, 99–108.

Healey, K. and Kennedy, R. (1993) Which families benefit from inpatient psychotherapeutic work at the Cassel Hospital? *British Journal of Psychotherapy,* 9, 394–404.

Hinshelwood, R. (1988) Psychotherapy in an inpatient setting. *Current Opinion in Psychiatry,* 1, 304–308.

James, O. (1986) The role of the nurse-therapist relationship in the therapeutic community. *International Review of Psycho-Analysis,* 11, 151–159.

Jones, M. (1952) *Social Psychiatry.* London: Tavistock.

Kernberg, O.F. (1984) *Severe Personality Disorders: Psychotherapeutic Strategies.* London: Yale University Press.

Knight, R. (1953) Management and psychotherapy of the borderline schizophrenic patient. *Bulletin of the Menninger Clinic,* 17, 139–150.

Main, T. (1957) The Ailment. *British Journal of Medical Psychology*, 30, 129–145. Reprinted T. Main (1989) *The Ailment and other Psycho-Analytic Essays.* London: Free Association Books.

Main, T. (1983) 'The concept of the therapeutic community: its variations and vicissitudes.' In M. Pines, ed. *The Evolution of Group Analysis.* London: Routledge & Regan Paul. Reprinted: Main, T. (1989) *The Ailment and other Psycho-Analytic Essays.* London: Free Association Books.

Masterson, J.F. (1972) *Treatment of the Borderline Adolescent: A Developmental Approach.* New York: Wiley.

Miller, L.J. (1989) Inpatient management of borderline personality disorder a review and update. *Journal of Personality Disorders*, 3, 122–134.

Norton, K.R.W. (1992a) Health of the Nation: The impact of personality disorder on 'key areas'. *Postgraduate Medical Journal*, 68, 350–354.

Norton, K.R.W. (1992b) A culture of enquiry: its preservation or loss. *International Journal of Therapeutic Communities*, 13, 3–26.

Norton, K.R.W. and Smith, S. (1994) *Problems with Patients: Managing Complicated Clinical Transactions* Cambridge: Cambridge University Press.

Norton, K.R.W. and Dolan, B. (1995a) Acting out and the institutional response. *Journal of Forensic Psychiatry*, 6, 317–332.

Norton, K.R.W. and Dolan, B. (1995b) Assessing change in personality disorder. *Current Opinion in Psychiatry*, 8, 371–375.

Pines, M. (1978) Group analytic psychotherapy with borderline personality disorder. *Group Analysis*, 11, 115–126.

Powell, G., Caan, W. and Crowe, M. (1994) What events precede violent incidents in psychiatric hospitals? *British Journal of Psychiatry*, 165, 107–112.

Schwartz, D., Flinn, D. and Slawson, P. (1974) Treatment of the suicidal character. *American Journal of Psychotherapy*, 28, 194–207.

Stanton, A.H. and Schwartz, M.S. (1954) *The Mental Hospital.* New York: Basic Books.

Stein, G. (1992) Drug treatment of the personality disorders. *British Journal of Psychiatry*, 161, 167–184.

Stone, M.H. (1993) Long-term outcome in personality disorder. *British Journal of Psychiatry*, 162, 299–313.

Tischler, L. (1986) 'Nurse/therapist supervision.' In R. Kennedy, ed. *The Family as In-Patient.* London: Free Association Books. p.95–107.

Tyrer, P. (1988) *Personality Disorder, Diagnosis, Management and Care.* London: Wright.

Whiteley, S. (1970) The response of psychopaths to a therapeutic community. *British Journal of Psychiatry*, 166, 517–529.

16

The Concept of Boundaries in Clinical Practice: Theoretical and Risk-management Dimensions*

Thomas Gutheil and Glen O. Gabbard
1993

. . . .

Editors' reflections

The concept of professional boundaries is now receiving the attention that it deserves: partly as a move to improve the quality of our professional work, and partly in response to sad accounts of boundary violations by professionals. In present clinical practice, the term 'boundaries' is frequently heard, but what are boundaries? This question is complicated by the fact that individuals within a team may have different ideas about what 'defines' a boundary. We conceive boundaries as marking out our professional identity and role; boundary violations occur when we find ourselves out of role, and therefore into another non-professional identity. Professors Gutheil and Gabbard are international experts in this field, and this paper is an excellent introduction to any discussion of boundaries, and how to keep them. This is particularly relevant for therapists and practitioners working with personality disordered individuals, since such

* Originally published in *American Journal of Psychiatry*, *150*, 2, 188–196. Reprinted with permission from the *American Journal of Psychiatry* © 1993 American Psychiatric Association.

service users have the capacity to draw us out of role through the feelings they invoke. Even quite minor role departures can be the beginning of a process that ends in significant boundary violations. This paper would be a good basis for a seminar or workshop on professional boundaries.

Abstract

The authors systematically examine the concept of boundaries and boundary viola-tions in clinical practice, particularly as they relate to recent sexual misconduct litiga-tion. They selectively review the literature on the subject and identify critical areas that require explication in terms of harmful versus nonharmful boundary issues short of sexual misconduct. These areas include role; time; place and space; money; gifts, services, and related matters; clothing; language; self-disclosure and related matters; and physical contact. While broad guidelines are helpful, the specific impact of a par-ticular boundary crossing can only be assessed by careful attention to the clinical context. Heightened awareness of the concepts of boundaries, boundary crossings, and boundary violations will both improve patient care and contribute to effective risk management.

(Am J Psychiatry 1993; 150:188–196)

INTRODUCTION

Role boundaries may be crisp or flexible or fuzzy, depending on the role under consideration and on the cultural climate.

Ingram (1991)

The concept of boundaries, particularly in the sense of boundary crossings and boundary violations, has come under increased scrutiny in relation to the wave of sexual misconduct cases (Gutheil, 1989) arising in litigation, ethics committee hearings, and complaints to boards of licensure. Like many concepts in psychotherapy, such as "therapy," "transference," and "alliance," the term proves slippery on closer observation. The literature tends to focus on patient–therapist sexual misconduct (Stone, 1976) as an extreme violation and not on the wide variety of lesser and more complex boundary crossings, many of which are, at first glance, less obvious but pose difficulties of their own for clinicians.

Clinicians tend to feel that they understand the concept of boundaries instinctively, but using it in practice or explaining it to others is often challenging. This latter problem is rendered more difficult by the tendency of the legal system, particularly plaintiffs' attorneys, to apply it mechanistically: any boundary crossing is bad, wrong, and harmful. Empirical evidence suggests that boundary violations frequently accompany or precede sexual misconduct (Borys and Pope, 1989; Gabbard, 1989; Gutheil, 1989), but the violations themselves do not always constitute malpractice or misconduct or even bad technique. However, modern clinicians should be aware of three principles that govern the relationship among boundaries, boundary crossings, boundary violations, and sexual misconduct.

First, *sexual misconduct usually begins with relatively minor boundary violations,* which often show a crescendo pattern of increasing intrusion into the patient's space that culminates in sexual contact. A direct shift from talking to intercourse is quite rare; the "slippery slope" is the characteristic scenario. As Gabbard (1989) and Simon (1989) have pointed out, a common sequence involves a transition from last-name to first-name basis; then personal conversation intruding on the clinical work; then some body contact (e.g., pats on the shoulder, massages, progressing to hugs); then trips outside the office; then sessions during lunch, sometimes with alcoholic beverages; then dinner; then movies or other social events; and finally sexual intercourse.

Second, *not all boundary crossings or even boundary violations lead to or represent evidence of sexual misconduct.* A clear boundary violation from one ideological perspective may be standard professional practice from another. For example, the so-called "Christian psychiatry movement" might condone the therapist's attendance at a church service with one or more patients, and various group therapeutic approaches or therapeutic communities may involve inherent boundary violations, as when some behaviorist schools permit hiring patients in therapy to do work in the treatment setting. Bad training, sloppy practice, lapses of judgment, idiosyncratic treatment philosophies, regional variations, and social and cultural conditioning may all be reflected in behavior that violates boundaries but that may not necessarily lead to sexual misconduct, be harmful, or deviate from the relevant standard of care.

Third, despite this complexity, *fact finders*—civil or criminal juries, judges, ethics committees of professional organizations, or state licensing boards—*often believe that the presence of boundary violations (or even crossings) is presumptive evidence of, or corroborates allegations of, sexual misconduct.*

To summarize the foregoing more concisely, albeit metaphorically, smoke usually leads to fire; one can, however, find smoke where there is no fire, and yet fact finders may assume that where there's smoke, there's fire. This metaphor is not trivial. In a notorious Massachusetts case (in which the doctor accused of sexual misconduct was eventually exonerated), the Board of Registration in

Medicine, the state licensing authority, noted in the course of the process, "There was an undisputed level of intimacy between the two [patient and doctor] that supports the inference of sexual relations" (transcript of board proceedings, citation withheld). In its language here, the board clearly articulated its "inference" of fire from the "undisputed" presence of smoke. Moreover, recent court decisions suggest a trend toward findings of liability for boundary violations even in the absence of sexual contact (Jorgenson, 1991). On this basis, the risk-management value of avoiding even the appearance of boundary violations should be self-evident.

This communication has three goals: 1) to review the subject in order to define, describe, and illustrate the range of boundary issues, 2) to demonstrate that crossing certain boundaries may at times be salutary, at times neutral, and at times harmful, and 3) to suggest preventive and reparative measures for clinicians dealing with boundary violations in themselves and their patients.

DEFINITIONS

What is a boundary? Is it too amorphous, protean, and abstract to define at all? Should we take refuge by saying, as St. Augustine was supposed to have said about time, "Time? I know what time is, provided you do not ask me?"

Part of the difficulty encountered in defining appropriate boundaries can be related to the historical tradition that modern therapists have inherited. The great figures in the field gave out mixed messages on the issue. Freud, for example, used metaphors involving the opacity of a mirror and the dispassionate objectivity of a surgeon to describe the analyst's role, but his own behavior in the analytic setting did not necessarily reflect the abstinence and anonymity that he advocated in his writings. He sent patients postcards, lent them books, gave them gifts, corrected them when they spoke in a misinformed manner about his family members, provided them with extensive financial support in some cases, and on at least one occasion gave a patient a meal (Lipton, 1977). Moreover, the line between professional and personal relationships in Freud's analytic practice was difficult to pinpoint. During vacations he would analyze Ferenczi while walking through the countryside. In one of his letters to Ferenczi, which were often addressed "Dear Son," he indicated that during his holiday he planned to analyze him in two sessions a day but also invited him to share at least one meal with him each day (unpublished manuscript by A. Hoffer). For Freud the analytic relationship could be circumscribed by the time boundaries of the analytic sessions, and other relationships were possible outside the analytic hours. The most striking illustration of this conception of boundaries is Freud's analysis of his own daughter, Anna.

Freud was not alone in establishing ambiguous analytic boundaries. When Melanie Klein was analyzing Clifford Scott, she encouraged him to follow her to the Black Forest for her holiday. Each day during this vacation, Scott underwent analysis for a 2-hour session while reclining on Klein's bed in her hotel room (Grosskurth, 1986). D.W. Winnicott, another therapist of considerable stature, occasionally took young patients into his home as part of his treatment of them (Winnicott, 1943). In Margaret Little's report of her analysis with Little (1990), she recalled how Winnicott held her hands clasped between his through many hours as she lay on the couch in a near-psychotic state. On one occasion he told her about another patient of his who had committed suicide and went into considerable detail about his countertransference reactions to the patient. He also ended each session with coffee and biscuits. These boundary transgressions by highly revered figures have occasionally been cited in ethics hearings as justification for unethical behavior. We wish to stress that these behaviors are no longer acceptable practice regardless of their place in the history of our field.

The problem of the contradiction between what the master therapists wrote and how they actually behaved in the clinical setting was compounded because psychoanalysis and psychotherapy are treatments that occur in a highly private context. The boundaries of the therapeutic relationship and the characteristics of acceptable technique were thus highly subjective and lacked standardization. This lack of clarity was partially addressed by Eissler's classic paper (1953) in which he suggested that in the ideal situation, the analyst's activity should be confined to interpretation. Any deviation from that model technique was defined by Eissler as a parameter. As examples of parameters, he cited Freud's setting a termination date for the Wolf Man and proposed a hypothetical situation in which an analyst might command a phobic patient to expose himself to the feared situation. By this standard of technique, Freud's own behavior, such as offering a meal to the Rat Man, has been regarded as indicative of an earlier technique that Freud subsequently abandoned (Zetzel, 1966) or a human failing rather than a technical recommendation (Shapiro, 1984).

Lipton (1977) took a strikingly different view of Freud's apparently unorthodox behavior with the Rat Man. He insisted that Freud's providing a meal for the patient should not be considered part of his psychoanalytic technique. Instead, it should be regarded as part of the nontechnical personal relationship that Freud had with this patient. He pointed out that in every analysis, the analyst is called upon to offer assistance in a personal way from time to time.

While the ramifications and fantasies produced by such behavior should be thoroughly analyzed, it would be erroneous, in Lipton's view, to expand the concept of technique to include all aspects of the analyst's relationship with the patient. Lipton expressed the following concern: "Modern technique tends to move from the position from which the analyst's technique is judged according to his purpose to one from which the analyst's technique is judged according to his behavior" (1977, p.262). He pointed out that following Eissler's model of analytic technique in its literal terms would cause any noninterpretive comment or action on the part of the analyst to be construed as a parameter.

Another major problem with any attempt to derive definitions of boundaries from psychoanalytic concepts of technique is that technique changes with treatments that are less expressive than analysis. As one moves along the expressive-supportive continuum of psychotherapy (Gabbard, 1990), one relies less on interpretation and more on alternative interventions such as clarification, confrontation, advice and praise, suggestion, and affirmation. Similarly, partial gratification of transference wishes is associated with supportive psychotherapy, whereas it is generally eschewed in psychoanalysis or highly expressive psychotherapy. Hence, there may be a built-in confusion between the notion of therapeutic boundaries and adjusting the technique to the ego organization of the patient.

Another approach to defining therapeutic boundaries is to conceptualize a therapeutic frame (Langs, 1976; Spruiell, 1983), i.e., an envelope or membrane around the therapeutic role that defines the characteristics of the therapeutic relationship. The analyst or therapist constructs the elements of the frame partly consciously and partly unconsciously. These elements include the regular scheduling of appointments, the duration of the appointments, arrangements for payment of the fee, and the office setting itself.

Does the patient's role have a boundary? Spruiell (1983) has noted that although the frame is deliberately unbalanced, the patient invariably joins the analyst in elaborating the frame. Most clinicians would agree, basing this answer on recollected violations they have witnessed, such as the patient who refers to the therapist as "Shrinkie" or springs from the chair and tries without warning to sit on the therapist's lap. It is clear, however, that the patient's boundary is a more forgiving and flexible one. The patient cannot be stopped from calling the therapist names, and that is part of the therapeutic process. The patient can be late and that can be discussed, but the therapist should not be late, and so on. In any case our focus here is on the clinician's boundary.

Let us also agree that the role of therapist embraces the structural aspects of therapy in addition to the content; these include time, place, and money, which may, together with other aspects discussed below, represent possible sites for boundary crossings or violations to occur. If this exploration is to be useful, we should adopt the convention that "boundary crossing" in this article is a descriptive term, neither laudatory nor pejorative. An assessor could then determine the impact of a boundary crossing on a case-by-case basis that takes into account the context and situation-specific facts, such as the possible harmfulness of this crossing to this patient. A violation, then, represents a *harmful* crossing, a transgression, of a boundary. An example might be the case of a patient who had experienced severe or traumatic boundary violations in childhood and who might consequently be highly sensitive to later violations, even those usually considered benign. Note also that the difference between a harmful and a nonharmful boundary crossing may lie in whether it is discussed or discussable; clinical exploration of a violation often defuses its potential for harm.

To organize the discussion we consider the matter of boundaries, boundary crossings, and boundary violations under a series of headings: role; time; place and space; money; gifts, services, and related matters; clothing; language; self-disclosure and related matters; and physical contact. Sexual misconduct as an extreme boundary violation has been extensively addressed elsewhere (Appelbaum and Gutheil, 1991; Gabbard, 1990; Gutheil, 1989; Simon, 1989) and is not separately reviewed here. We should also point out that in addition to serving as antecedents to sexual misconduct, some of these areas of boundary crossing may represent ethical violations in and of themselves.

Role

Role boundaries constitute the essential boundary issue. To conceptualize this entity, one might ask, "Is this what a therapist does?" Although subject to ideological variations, this touchstone question not only identifies the question of clinical role but serves as a useful orienting device for avoiding the pitfalls of role violations.

> A middle-aged borderline patient, attempting to convey how deeply distressed she felt about her situation, leaped from her chair in the therapist's office and threw herself to her knees at the therapist's feet, clasping his hand in both of her own and crying, "Do you understand how awful it's been for me?" The therapist said gently, "You know, this is really interesting, what's happening here—but it isn't therapy; please go back to your chair." The patient did so, and the incident was explored verbally.

Although such limit setting may appear brusque to some clinicians, it may be the only appropriate response to halt boundary-violating "acting in" (especially of the impulsive or precipitous kind) and to make the behavior available for analysis as part of the therapy.

Almost all patients who enter into a psychotherapeutic process struggle with the unconscious wish to view the therapist as the ideal parent who, unlike the real parents, will gratify all their childhood wishes (Viederman, 1991). As a result of the longings stirred up by the basic transference situation of psycho-therapy or psychoanalysis, it is imperative that some degree of abstinence be maintained (Novey, 1991). However, strict abstinence is neither desirable nor possible, and total frustration of all the patient's wishes creates a powerful influence on the patient in its own right (Lipton, 1977; Viederman, 1991).

In attempting to delineate the appropriate role for the therapist vis-à-vis the patient's wishes and longings to be loved and held, it is useful to differentiate between "libidinal demands," which cannot be gratified without entering into ethical transgressions and damaging enactments, and "growth needs," which prevent growth if not gratified to some extent (Casement, 1990). Greenson (1967) made a similar distinction when he noted that the rule of abstinence was constructed to avoid the gratification of a patient's neurotic and infantile wishes, not to lead to a sterile form of treatment in which all the patient's wishes are frustrated.

Efforts to delineate the two varieties of needs often lead to problems in the area of defining the appropriate role for the therapist. Certainly, the patient may have legitimate wishes to be empathically understood, but when the therapist goes too far in the direction of trying to provide parental functions that were not supplied by the original parents, the patient may experience the therapist as making false promises. Casement (1990) expressed reservations about Freud's providing a meal to the Rat Man because of the possibility that the patient may have experienced Freud's taking responsibility for a particular part of his life as an implicit promise that Freud was prepared to take over responsibility for other areas of the patient's life as well. Clearly, a therapist cannot become the "good mother" or "good father" in a literal sense and attempt to make up for all the deprivations of childhood. Even when therapists feel as though they are being coerced into a parental role by their patients, they must strive not to conform to the patients' expectations. Spruiell (1983) made the following observation: "It is as disastrous for analysts to actually treat their patients like children as it is for analysts to treat their own children as patients" (p.12).

The therapist's role is subject to some variation, of course. While most therapy is talking, there may be times when it is appropriate, for example, to write a letter on a patient's behalf. Under some circumstances, such a "breach of the frame" (Langs, 1976) might constitute a boundary violation, as when the therapist attempts to intervene in some extra-therapeutic realm of the patient's life (e.g., a therapist wrote a stern letter to a patient's employer rebuking the latter for giving the patient excessively burdensome tasks on the job). In addition, since different modalities of therapy are commonly combined, the "talking therapist" might appropriately give medications, conceivably by injection at times—a clear boundary crossing but presumably therapeutic and benign.

Time

Time is, of course, a boundary, defining the limits of the session itself while providing structure and even containment for many patients, who derive reassurance because they will have to experience the various stresses of reminiscing, reliving, and so forth for a set time only. The beginnings and endings of sessions—starting or stopping late or early—are both susceptible to crossings of this boundary. Such crossings may be subtle or stark.

A male psychiatrist came in to the hospital to see his female inpatient for marathon sessions at odd times, such as from 2:00 to 6:00 in the morning, rationalizing that this procedure was dictated by scheduling problems. This relationship eventually became overtly sexual.

An interesting prejudice about violating the boundary of time has evolved in sexual misconduct cases, a prejudice deriving from the fact that a clinician interested in having a sexual relationship with a patient might well schedule that patient for the last hour of the day (although, of course, after-work time slots have always been popular). In the fog of uncertainty surrounding sexual misconduct (usually a conflict of credibilities without witnesses), this factor has gleamed with so illusory a brightness that some attorneys seem to presume that because the patient had the last appointment of the day, sexual misconduct occurred! Short of seeing patients straight through the night, this problem does not seem to have a clear solution. Admittedly, however, from a risk-management standpoint, a patient in the midst of an intense erotic transference to the therapist might best be seen, when possible, during high-traffic times when other people (e.g., secretaries, receptionists, and even other patients) are around.

Langs (1982) noted that the boundary of time may be psychologically violated when the therapist brings up material from a previous session. Some patients, indeed, feel that this practice is disruptive and is a departure by the therapist from the here and now. However, most clinicians would regard this view as extreme, since effective therapy depends on continuity from session to session.

The issue of the appropriateness of phone calls between psychotherapy sessions is a controversial one, particularly when the patient suffers from borderline personality disorder. Some therapists view such phone calls as necessary and expectable in light of the borderline patient's difficulties with evocative memory (Alder, 1985; Alder and Buie, 1979). In other words, the patient's inability to evoke a holding, soothing introject causes anxiety of catastrophic proportions related to the fear that the therapist has disappeared. Phone calls are a way of reestablishing contact with the therapist and soothing this anxiety, which might otherwise lead to ill-advised self-destructive behavior. On the other hand, other therapists view such calls as unnecessary and countertherapeutic (Adler, 1985; Adler and Buie, 1979). These therapists go to great lengths in the initial contractual period, at the beginning of therapy, to extract an agreement from the patient that phone calls will be used only in emergency situations. This controversy reflects how a boundary violation may be defined according to the extent to which the appropriate treatment is viewed as having an expressive versus a supportive emphasis.

Place and space

The therapist's office or a room on a hospital unit is obviously the locale for almost all therapy; some exceptions are noted in the next section. Exceptions usually constitute boundary crossings but are not always harmful. Some examples include accompanying a patient to court for a hearing, visiting a patient at home, and seeing a patient in the intensive care unit after an overdose or in jail after an arrest.

Some boundary crossings of place can have a constructive effect. As with medication, the timing and dosage are critical:

> After initially agreeing to attend his analysand's wedding, the analyst later declined, reasoning that his presence would be inappropriately distracting. Later, after the death of the analysand's first child, he attended the funeral service. Both his absence at the first occasion and his presence at the second were felt as helpful and supportive by the analysand. They both agreed later that the initial plan to attend the wedding was an error.

A relevant lesson from this example is that boundary violations can be reversed or undone with further consideration and discussion. At times, an apology by the therapist is appropriate and even necessary.

Some sexual misconduct cases reveal space violations that seem to manifest wishes for fusion on the part of the therapist, as in the following case:

A lesbian therapist treating a female patient would contrive to use the bathroom at the clinic whenever the patient did so and, entering the adjoining stall, would attempt to continue the conversation. The relationship became overtly and exploitatively sexual, with the therapist often wearing the patient's clothes to work the next day after they had spent the night together.

Sorties out of the office usually merit special scrutiny. While home visits were a central component of the community psychiatry movement, the shift in the professional climate is such that the modern clinician is best advised to perform this valuable service with an opposite-sex chaperon and to document the event in some detail.

Sessions during lunch are an extremely common form of boundary violation. This event appears to be a common way station along the path of increasing boundary crossings culminating in sexual misconduct. Although clinicians often advance the claim that therapy is going on, so, inevitably, is much purely social behavior; it does not *look* like therapy, at least to a jury. Lunch sessions are not uncommonly followed by sessions during dinner, then just dinners, then other dating behavior, eventually including intercourse. Sessions in cars represent another violation of place. Typically, the clinician gives the patient a ride home under various circumstances. Clinician and patient then park (e.g., in front of the patient's house) and finish up the presumably therapeutic conversation. From a fact finder's viewpoint, many exciting things happen in cars, but therapy is usually not one of them.

The complexity of the matter increases, however, when we consider other therapeutic ideologies. For example, it would not be a boundary violation for a behaviorist, under certain circumstances, to accompany a patient in a car, to an elevator, to an airplane, or even to a public restroom (in the treatment of paruresis, the fear of urinating in a public restroom) as part of the treatment plan for a particular phobia. The existence of a body of professional literature, a clinical rationale, and risk-benefit documentation will be useful in protecting the clinician in such a situation from misconstruction of the therapeutic efforts.

Money

Money is a boundary in the sense of defining the business nature of the therapeutic relationship. This is not love, it's work. Indeed, some would argue that the fee received by the therapist is the only appropriate and allowable material gratification to be derived from clinical work (Epstein and Simon, 1990). Patient and clinician may each have conflicts about this distinction (Krueger,

1986), but consultative experience makes clear that trouble begins precisely when the therapist stops thinking of therapy as work.

On the other hand, most clinicians learned their trade by working with indigent patients and feel that some attempt should be made to pay back this debt by seeing some patients for free—a form of "tithing," if you will. Note that this *decision*—to see a patient for free and to discuss that with the patient—is quite different from simply letting the billing lapse or allowing the debt to mount. The latter examples are boundary crossings, perhaps violations.

Consultative experience also suggests that the usual problem underlying a patient's mounting debt is the clinician's conflict about money and its dynamic meanings. Initially reluctant to bring up the unpaid bill, the clinician may soon become too angry to discuss it. Explorations of the dynamic meaning of the bill are more convincing when they do not take place through clenched teeth. A clinician stuck at this countertransference point may simply let it slide. In the minds of fact finders, this raises a question: "The clinician seems curiously indifferent to making a living; could the patient be paying in some other currency?"—a line of speculation one does not wish to foster.

In rural areas even today, payments to physicians may take the form of barter: when the doctor delivers your child, you pay with two chickens and the new calf. For the dynamic therapist this practice poses some problems, because it blurs the boundary between payment and gift (covered in the next section). The clinician should take a case at a reasonable fee or make a *decision* to see the patient for a low fee (e.g., one dollar) or none. Barter is confusing and probably ill-advised today. Of course, all such decisions require documentation.

Gifts, services, and related matters

A client became very upset during an interview with her therapist and began to cry. The therapist, proffering a tissue, held out a hand-tooled Florentine leather case in which a pocket pack of tissues had been placed. After the patient had withdrawn a tissue, the therapist impulsively said, "Why don't you keep the case?" In subsequent supervision the therapist came to understand that this "gift" to the patient was an unconscious bribe designed to avert the anger that the therapist sensed just below the surface of the patient's sorrow.

This gift was also a boundary violation, placing unidentified obligations on the patient and constituting a form of impulsive acting in. A related boundary violation is the use of favors or services from the patient for the benefit of the therapist, as Simon's startling vignette illustrates:

> Within a few months of starting…psychotherapy, the patient was return-
> ing the therapist's library books for him "as a favor.".… The patient began

having trouble paying her treatment bill, so she agreed—at the therapist's suggestion—to clean the therapist's office once a week in partial payment... The patient also agreed to get the therapist's lunch at a nearby delicatessen before each session (1989, p.106).

The obvious exploitive nature of these boundary violations destroys even the semblance of therapy for the patient's benefit.

When Freud heard that one of his patients was planning to buy a set of his complete works, he gave the patient the set as a gift (Blanton, 1971). Immediately following the receipt of this gift, Freud's patient found that he was unable to use his dreams productively in the analysis as he had before. Freud related this "drying up" to the gift and noted, "You will see from this what difficulties gifts in analysis always make" (p.42).

Other boundary crossings can be relatively minor but can promote a chain of subsequent crossings, as in this example:

A patient walked into the room while her therapist was pouring coffee from a carafe. He later described how he had felt socially incapable of not offering some coffee to the patient and had indeed offered some. At the next session, the patient brought doughnuts.

As the vignette shows, many boundary problems may arise at the interface between manners and technique. In contrast to the potentially harmful or at least confusing effects of the preceding examples, compare the practice (not uncommon among psychopharmacologists) of giving patients, as part of treatment, educational texts designed for laypersons (e.g., giving *Mood-swing* (Feive, 1976) to a patient with bipolar disorder). Such a boundary crossing may foster mastery of the illness through information—a positive result. A similar point might be made for judicious "gifts" of medication samples for indigent patients. These two instances represent clear boundary crossings that have some justification. Ideally, even these should be discussed with an ear to any possible negative effects:

A patient in long-term therapy had struggled for years with apparent infertility and eventually, with great difficulty, arranged for adoption of a child. Two years later she unexpectedly conceived and finally gave birth. Her therapist, appreciating the power and meaning of this event, sent congratulatory flowers to the hospital.

In this case, the therapist followed social convention in a way that—though technically a boundary crossing—represented a response appropriate to the real relationship. Offering a tissue to a crying patient and expressing condolences to a bereaved one are similar examples of appropriate responses outside the classic boundaries of the therapeutic relationship.

Clothing

Clothing represents a social boundary the transgression of which is usually inappropriate to the therapeutic situation, yet a patient may appropriately be asked to roll up a sleeve to permit measurement of blood pressure. Excessively revealing or frankly seductive clothing worn by the therapist may represent a boundary violation with potentially harmful effects to patients, but the issue can also be overdone, as in the following case:

> A patient in a western state, as part of a sexual misconduct allegation that a jury later found to be false, accused the therapist (among other things) of conducting therapy sessions with the top two buttons of his shirt undone. While such a phenomenon might conceivably represent a violation for a very sensitive patient, evidence was introduced that revealed the exaggerated nature of this claim in *this* case.

Berne (1972) noted the technical error of the male clinician who, confronting a patient whose skirt was pulled up high, began to explain to the patient his sexual fantasies in response to this event. Berne suggested instead saying to the patient, "Pull your skirt down." Similar directness of limit setting appears to be suited to the patient who—either from psychosis or the wish to provoke—begins to take off her clothes in the office. As before, the comment, "This behavior is inappropriate, and it isn't therapy; please put your clothes back on," said in a calm voice, is a reasonable response.

Language

As part of the otherwise laudable efforts to humanize and demystify psychiatry a few decades back, the use of a patient's first name was very much in vogue. While this may indeed convey greater warmth and closeness, such usage is a two-edged sword. There is always the possibility that patients may experience the use of first names as misrepresenting the professional relationship as a social friendship (Epstein and Simon, 1990). There may well be instances when using first names is appropriate, but therapists must carefully consider whether they are creating a false sense of intimacy that may subsequently backfire:

> A middle-aged woman tried for more than a year to get her therapist to use her first name, but the requests were denied, and exploration of the issue took place instead. After some time the patient recovered memories of pre-

viously repressed material, in part because of increased trust in the therapist. The patient spontaneously related her trust to the use of last names as
a boundary issue; boundaries had been badly blurred in her family and
this had included sexual abuse.

There are distinct advantages to addressing the adult in the patient, in terms of
fostering the adult observing ego for the alliance. Trainees often do not see the
paradox of expecting adult behavior on the ward from someone they themselves call "Jimmy," which is what people called the patient when he was much
younger. Last names also emphasize that this process is work or business, an
atmosphere which may promote a valuable mature perspective and minimize
acting out. In addition, calling someone by the name used by primary objects
may foster transference perceptions of the therapist when they are not
desirable, as with a borderline patient prone to forming severe psychotic
transferences. For balance, however, recall that use of last names may also sound
excessively distant, formal, and aloof.

Tone is also a part of language. A patient won a settlement in an allegation
of sexual misconduct when the tape recording she had made of a phone call
from her therapist revealed his intimate, seductive tone. The therapist's attorney
urged the settlement for fear that the jury would hear the intimate tone as
evidence of a sexual relationship.

Word choice can also be violative, as when the therapist inquires, "What are
you feeling now in your vagina?" Note that this inquiry might be proper in
analytic therapy after appropriate preparation. Clinical utility aside, the way in
which such explorations may violate boundaries should be kept in mind.

Finally, psychotherapy may be a forum for sadomasochistic enactments in
which aggressive verbal abuse grows out of countertransference sadism. Cruel
and contemptuous comments by the therapist may be rationalized as therapeutic confrontation.

Self-disclosure and related matters

Few clinicians would argue that the therapist's self-disclosure is always a
boundary crossing. Psychoanalysis and intensive psychotherapy involve
intense personal relationships. A useful therapeutic alliance may be forged by
the therapist's willingness to acknowledge that a painful experience of the
patient is familiar to himself (Viederman, 1991). However, when a therapist
begins to indulge in even mild forms of self-disclosure, it is an indication for
careful self-scrutiny regarding the motivations for departure from the usual
therapeutic stance. Gorkin (1987) observed that many therapists harbor a wish
to be known by their patients as a "real person," especially as the termination of

the therapy approaches. While it may be technically correct for a therapist to become more spontaneous at the end of the therapeutic process, therapists who become more self-disclosing as the therapy ends must be sure that their reasons for doing so are not related to their own unfulfilled needs in their private lives but, rather, are based on an objective assessment that increased focus on the real relationship is useful for the patient in the termination process.

Self-disclosure, however, represents a complex issue. Clearly, therapists may occasionally use a neutral example from their own lives to illustrate a point. Sharing the impact of a borderline patient's behavior on the therapist may also be useful. The therapist's self-revelation, however, of personal fantasies or dreams; of social, sexual, or financial details; of specific vacation plans; or of expected births or deaths in the family is usually burdening the patient with information, whereas it is the patient's fantasies that might best be explored. The issue is somewhat controversial: a number of patients (and, surprisingly, some therapists) believe that the patient is somehow entitled to this kind of information. In any case, it is a boundary violation and as such may be used by the legal system to advance or support a claim of sexual misconduct. The reasoning is that the patient knows so much about the therapist's personal life that they must have been intimate (compare the remark by a board of registration, quoted earlier).

Subtler variations on the information theme may occur, as when a therapist sees members of a couple in parallel treatment but separately alludes in one member's session to material from the other's. Sensitivity in this area may run quite high:

> A patient had a dream involving Nazis. In the interpretation the therapist suggested that this detail referred to himself. The patient seemed doubtful. The therapist noted that the interpretation was based in part on the fact that other patients of his had dreamed of Nazis in response to the therapist's German last name. The patient's mood changed; only later was she able to tell the therapist how violated she had felt at his "intruding" other patients into the session.

Although the intrusion was at a verbal level only, the impact was clear for this patient, who had been subjected to some disregard of her boundaries in previous therapy.

Finally, the boundary can be violated from the other side. An example would be the therapist's using data from the therapy session for personal gain, such as insider information on stock trading, huge profits to be made in real estate, and the like.

Physical contact

To place the issue of physical contact in context, it should be noted that psychiatrists traditionally performed their own physical examinations. This practice has declined so markedly that a senior psychiatrist recently wrote about examining a patient's bruised leg as a major return to the past. Hospitals commonly use internists for this purpose. Psychiatric residents still do their own physical examinations but commonly maintain distance by examining each other's patients. Abnormal Involuntary Movement Scale examinations for tardive dyskinesia are often the only routine physical contact.

There is room here for regrets. Physicians working with a patient with AIDS or HIV seropositivity often describe wishing to touch the patient in some benign manner (pat the back, squeeze an arm, pat a hand) in every session. They reason that such patients feel like lepers, and therapeutic touch is called for in these cases. But even such humane interventions must be scrutinized and, indeed, be documented to prevent their misconstruction in today's climate.

From the viewpoint of current risk-management principles, a handshake is about the limit of social physical contact at this time. Of course, a patient who attempts a hug in the last session after 7 years of intense, intensive, and successful therapy should probably not be hurled across the room. However, most hugs from patients should be discouraged in tactful, gentle ways by words, body language, positioning, and so forth. Patients who deliberately or provocatively throw their arms around the therapist despite repeated efforts at discouragement should be stopped. An appropriate response is to step back, catch both wrists in your hands, cross the patient's wrists in front of you, so that the crossed arms form a barrier between bodies, and say firmly, "Therapy is a talking relationship; please sit down so we can discuss your not doing this any more." If the work degenerates into grabbing, consider seriously termination and referral, perhaps to a therapist of a different gender.

What is one to make of the brands of therapy that include physical contact, such as Rolfing? Presumably, the boundary extends to that limited physical contact, and the patient expects it and grants consent; thus, no actual violation occurs. Massage therapists may struggle with similar issues, however. In other ideologies the issue may again be the impact of the appearance of a violation:

> A therapist—who claimed that her school of practice involved hugging her female patient at the beginning and end of every session, without apparent harm—eventually had to terminate therapy with the patient for noncompliance with the therapeutic plan. The enraged patient filed a sexual misconduct claim against the therapist. Despite the evidence showing that this claim was probably false (a specious suit triggered by

rage at the therapist), the insurer settled because of the likelihood that a jury would not accept the principle of "hug at the start and hug at the end but no hugs in between." If the claim was indeed false, this is a settlement based on boundary violations alone.

At another level this vignette nicely suggests how nonsexual boundary violations may be harmful to a patient in much the same way that actual sexual misconduct is. Instead of engaging the patient in a mourning process to deal with the resentment and grief about the deprivations of her childhood, the therapist who hugs a patient is often attempting to provide the physical contact normally offered by a parent. The patient then feels entitled to more demonstrations of caring and assumes that if gratification in the form of hugs is available, other wishes will be granted as well (compare Smith's (1977) concept of the "golden fantasy" that all needs will be met by therapy). When actual physical contact occurs, the crucial psychotherapeutic distinction between the symbolic and the concrete is lost (Casement, 1990), and the patient may feel that powerful infantile longings within will finally be satisfied.

CONCLUSIONS

Boundary crossings may be benign or harmful, may take many forms, and may pose problems related to both treatment and potential liability. The differences in impact may depend on whether clinical judgment has been used to make the decision, whether adequate discussion and exploration have taken place, and whether documentation adequately records the details. The complexity of the subject and the variability of results from case-by-case analysis merit empirical study. Educational materials are available through the Office of Public Affairs of the American Psychiatric Association. Heightened awareness of the concepts of boundaries, boundary crossings, and boundary violations will both improve patient care and contribute to effective risk management.

   In an effort to prevent more serious boundary violations of a sexual nature, Epstein and Simon (1990) have developed an exploitation index which comprises a list of questions that therapists can ask themselves about their current behavior with patients. In this manner these authors have attempted to provide an ongoing self-monitoring system. While such approaches may be useful for some clinicians, we must acknowledge that considerable personal variation exists in our field. The relationships between therapist and patient vary from one therapist to another, and there are even variations across patients in the practice of one therapist. As Lipton (1977) observed, it is ultimately impossible to codify or prescribe a personal relationship between therapist and patient in a precise manner. Perhaps the best risk management involves careful consideration of any departures from one's usual practice accompanied by careful documentation of the reasons for the departure. Finally, the value of consultation with a respected colleague should be a built-in part of every practitioner's risk-management program.

REFERENCES

Adler, G. (1985) *Borderline Psychopathology and Its Treatment*. New York: Jason Aronson.

Adler, G. and Buie, D.H. Jr (1979) Aloneness and borderline psychopathology: the possible relevance of child development issues. *International Journal of Psychoanalysis*, 60, 83–96.

Appelbaum, P.S. and Gutheil, T.G. (1991) *Clinical Handbook of Psychiatry and the Law*. 2nd ed. Baltimore: Williams and Wilkins.

Berne, E. (1972) *What Do You Say After You Say Hello? The Psychology of Human Destiny*. New York: Grove Press.

Blanton, S. (1971) *Diary of My Analysis With Sigmund Freud*. New York: Hawthorn Books.

Borys, D.S. and Pope K.S. (1989) Dual relationships between therapist and client: a national study of psychologists, psychiatrists, and social workers. *Professional Psychology: Research and Practice*, 20, 280–293.

Casement, P.J. (1990) The meeting of needs in psychoanalysis. *Psychoanalytic Inquiry*, 10, 325–346.

Eissler, K.R. (1953) The effect of the structure of the ego on psychoanalytic technique. *Journal of the American Psychoanalytic Association*, 1, 104–143.

Epstein, R.S. and Simon, R.I. (1990) The exploitation index: an early warning indicator of boundary violations in psychotherapy. *Bulletin of the Menninger Clinic*, 54, 450–465.

Fieve, R. (1976) *Moodswing: The Third Revolution in Psychiatry*. New York: Bantam Books.

Gabbard, G.O. (ed) (1989) *Sexual Exploitation in Professional Relationships*. Washington, DC: American Psychiatric Press.

Gabbard, G.O. (1990) *Psychodynamic Psychiatry in Clinical Practice*. Washington, DC: American Psychiatric Press.

Gorkin, M. (1987) *The Uses of Countertransference*. Northvale, NJ: Jason Aronson.

Greenson, R.R. (1967) *The Technique of Psychoanalysis, vol 1*. New York: International Universities Press.

Grosskurth, P. (1986) *Melanie Klein: Her World and Her Work*. New York: Alfred A Knopf.

Gutheil, T.G. (1989) Borderline personality disorder, boundary violations, and patient-therapist sex: Medicolegal pitfalls. *American Journal of Psychiatry*, 146, 597–602.

Ingram, D.H. (1991) Intimacy in the psychoanalytic relationship: a preliminary sketch. *American Journal of Psychoanalysis*, 51, 403–411.

Jorgenson, L. (1991) Consultation forum. *Psychodynamic Letter*, 1 (10), 7–8.

Kernberg, O.F. (1984) *Severe Personality Disorders: Psychotherapeutic Strategies*. New Haven, Conn: Yale University Press.

Kernberg, O.F., Selzer, M.A., Koenigsberg, H.W., Carr, A.C., Appelbaum, H.A. (1989) *Psychodynamic Psychotherapy of Borderline Patients*. New York: Basic Books.

Krueger, D.W. (ed.) (1986) *The Last Taboo: Money As Symbol and Reality in Psychotherapy and Psychoanalysis*. New York: Brunner/ Mazel.

Langs, R. (1976) *The Bipersonal Field*. New York: Jason Aronson.

Langs, R. (1982) *Psychotherapy: A Basic Text.* New York: Jason Aronson.

Lipton, S.D. (1977) The advantages of Freud's technique as shown in his analysis of the Rat Man. *International Journal of Psychoanalysis,* 58, 255–273.

Little, M.I. (1990) *Psychotic Anxieties and Containment: A Personal Record of an Analysis with Winnicott.* Northvale, NJ: Jason Aronson.

Novey, R. (1991) The abstinence of the psychoanalyst. *Bulletin of the Menninger Clinic,* 55, 344–362.

Shapiro, T. (1984) On neutrality. *Journal of the American Psychoanalytic Association,* 32, 269–282.

Simon, R.I. (1989) Sexual exploitation of patients: how it begins before it happens. *Psychiatric Annals,* 19, 104–122.

Smith, S. (1977) The golden fantasy: a regressive reaction to separation anxiety. *International Journal of Psychoanalysis,* 58, 311–324.

Spruiell, V. (1983) The rules and frames of the psychoanalytic situation. *Psychoanalytic Quarterly,* 52, 1–33.

Stone, M.H. (1976) Boundary violations between therapist and patient. *Psychiatric Annals,* 6, 670–677.

Viederman, M. (1991) The real person of the analyst and his role in the process of psychoanalytic cure. *Journal of the American Psychoanalytic Association,* 39, 451–489.

Winnicott, D.W. (1943) Hate in the counter-transference. *International Journal of Psychoanalysis,* 30, 69–74.

Zetzel, E.R. (1966) Additional notes upon a case of obsessional neurosis: Freud 1909. *International Journal of Psychoanalysis,* 47, 123–129.

. . . .

Points for reflective practice

- What implications do these papers have for your clinical practice?

- How could the ideas generated from any of these papers become integrated into your own 'everyday' work with personality disorder? And within the team or organisation within which you work?

- As a staff group and individually, how do you understand and manage treatment 'failure' or 'sabotage'?

- What are your 'boundaries'? How do you maintain them at work?

- What does a 'boundary violation' mean to you? And to other staff whom you work with?

- Reflect upon your work with service users over the past week. Have there been occasions when boundaries have been challenged or crossed? How did you feel? How did you manage the scenario? How would other staff you work with manage the same situation? What can be done differently?

- What are your opportunities at work to maintain a reflective space within which to consider your relationships with service users and with colleagues?

. . . .

Contributors

Dr Gwen Adshead is a forensic psychiatrist and psychotherapist. She works at Broadmoor Hospital, Berkshire, UK. Email: gwen.adshead@wlmht.nhs.uk

Dr James A. Chu is Associate Professor of Psychiatry at Harvard University, USA. He has taught widely throughout the United States and internationally. As a teacher, Dr Chu is known for his empathic and pragmatic approach to understanding and treating survivors of childhood abuse. His publications in the psychiatric literature include basic research on the effects of childhood abuse and discussions concerning the nature and techniques of treatment of abuse survivors. He is the author of the 1998 book *Rebuilding Shattered Lives*. Dr Chu is a fellow of the American Psychiatric Association, and a fellow and a past president of the International Society for the Study of Dissociation.

Dr Michael Craft (1928–2004) was Consultant Psychiatrist and Superintendent of the North Wales Adolescent Unit in Conway, UK. He published several research studies on the origins of psychopathy in delinquent youth.

Marcus Evans has a background in nursing and is a psychoanalytic psychotherapist at the Maudsley Psychotherapy Unit, London. He is affiliated with the Tavistock Clinic, London, including working as a senior lecturer there. He is a member of the Association for Psychoanalytic Psychotherapy in the NHS.

Dr Glen O. Gabbard graduated from Rush Medical College, Chicago and completed his residency at the Karl Menninger School of Psychiatry, Topeka, Kansas, USA. He worked at the Menninger Clinic for 26 years, spending 5 years as Director of the Menninger Hospital and 7 years as the Bessie Walker Callaway Distinguished Professor of Psychoanalysis and Education at the Karl Menninger School of Psychiatry. He has also served as Director of the Topeka Institute for Psychoanalysis. Dr Gabbard moved to Baylor College of Medicine in 2001, where he is now Brown Foundation Chair of Psychoanalysis and Professor of Psychiatry, as well as Director of the Baylor Psychiatry Clinic. Dr Gabbard has received many awards, including the American Psychiatric Association Adolf Meyer Award in 2004 and that same organisation's Distinguished Service Award in 2002. He has authored or edited 20 books and over 250 papers. Dr Gabbard is currently the joint Editor-in-Chief of the International Journal of Psychoanalysis and Associate Editor of the American Journal of Psychiatry. He is a training and supervising analyst at the Houston/Galveston Psychoanalytic Institute.

Sir William Clive Granger retired from his post as Emeritus Professor at the University of California, San Diego in 2003. He was awarded the 2003 Nobel Memorial Prize in economic sciences. He was awarded the dignity of Knight Bachelor in the New Year's honours list in 2005.

Dr James E. Groves is a psychiatrist at Massachusettes General Hospital and an associate professor at Harvard University.

Dr Thomas G. Gutheil is Professor of Psychiatry in the Department of Psychiatry, Beth Israel-Deaconess Medical Center, Harvard Medical School, USA. Dr Gutheil has been previously associated with the Massachusetts Mental Health Center, Boston, for more than a third of a century and had served as a staff member there for 34 years. An internationally known teacher, lecturer, author and consultant on medico-legal issues, risk management and malpractice prevention, Dr Gutheil is the first professor of psychiatry in the history of the Harvard Medical School to be board certified in both general and forensic psychiatry. He was the year 2000 President of the American Academy of Psychiatry and Law, the National Forensic Psychiatric Association, and is the current President of the International Academy of Law and Mental Health. In total, Dr Gutheil has been author or co-author of over 250 articles, books or book chapters in the national and international clinical and forensic literature as well as several teaching audiotapes and videotapes.

Dr Scott Henderson is an emeritus professor of Psychiatry at The Australian National University. He is a graduate in medicine from Aberdeen, Scotland, and a practicing clinician whose research career has been in the epidemiology of mental disorders. He recognises the relevance of primate evolution in many aspects of human behaviour. The concept of care-eliciting emerged from the seminal work of John Bowlby's attachment theory. Its relevance can be seen in both everyday life, at all ages, as well as in mental illness. Scott Henderson lives in Canberra, Australia. He is Associate Editor of the Australian and New Zealand Journal of Psychiatry.

Dr R.D. Hinshelwood is a member of the British Psychoanalytical Society, and currently holds the post of Professor of Psychoanalysis at the Centre for Psychoanalytic Studies, University of Essex, UK. He is a fellow of the Royal College of Psychiatrists, and previously was Clinical Director of the Cassell Hospital in Richmond. He is a past Chair of the Association of Therapeutic Communities. Professor Hinshelwood has written extensively on psychoanalysis and founded the International Journal of Therapeutic Communities (now Therapeutic Communities) in 1980 and the British Journal of Psychotherapy in 1984

Thomas Forrest Main (1911–1990) was best known for founding the therapeutic community at the Cassell Hospital, Surrey, UK. He was a psychoanalyst who worked with both individuals and groups.

Professor Gethin Morgan is an emeritus professor of Psychiatry at Bristol University.

Dr Kingsley Norton is Head of Psychotherapy, St Bernard's Hospital, Middlesex, UK. From 1989 to 2006 he was the director of Henderson Hospital in Surrey, England. He is a Jungian analyst and has previously published three books on how to deal with patients who are difficult to treat. He is the author of over 80 articles and chapters, many in the field of personality disorder.

Geoffrey Stephenson is now Emeritus Professor of Social Psychology at the University of Kent. He has published widely in the fields of experimental social psychology, organisational psychology and legal and crimonological psychology.

Professor George Vaillant is a psychiatrist at Harvard Medical School. He is Director of the Study of Adult Development at the Harvard University Health Service and the author of numerous books and research studies on the development of the personality across the life span.

Darryl Watts is a consultant adult psychiatrist whose last place of work was Handley Cross House, Hertfordshire.

Dr Mary Whittle is a consultant forensic psychiatrist at the John Howard Centre in London.

Dr Donald Winnicott (1896–1971) was a paediatrician and psychoanalyst, who worked with disturbed children and their mothers during the Second World War. For an excellent biography, see *D.W. Winnicott: A Biographical Portrait* by Brett Kahr (London: Karnac, 1996).

EDITORS

Dr Gwen Adshead is Consultant Forensic Psychotherapist at Broadmoor Hospital. She trained first as a forensic psychiatrist before training as group analyst at the Institute of Group Analysis. Gwen has a research interest in attachment theory applied to forensic psychiatry and in the group dynamics of forensic organisations.

Dr Caroline Jacob is in her third year of higher specialist psychiatric training in forensic psychotherapy. She currently works in both psychotherapy and forensic psychiatry in Bristol, UK, in addition to some sessional experience in the forensic psychotherapy department at Broadmoor Hospital.

Subject Index

Author Index